HEALTH EVALUATION
an entry to the health care system

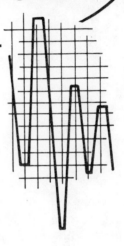

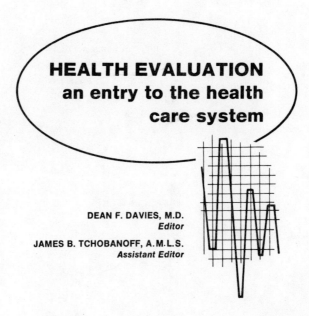

HEALTH EVALUATION
an entry to the health care system

DEAN F. DAVIES, M.D.
Editor

JAMES B. TCHOBANOFF, A.M.L.S.
Assistant Editor

Selected topics from the Third Annual Meeting of the Society for Advanced Medical Systems at Memphis, Tennessee.

Symposia Specialists
MEDICAL BOOKS

 INTERCONTINENTAL MEDICAL BOOK CORPORATION
381 Park Avenue South, New York, New York 10016 and London

Library of Congress Catalog
Card No. 73-82039

ISBN 0-88372-016-7

Contents

PLENARY SESSION I

The Engineer and Advanced Medical Systems   1
Lester Goodman, Ph.D.
Chief, Biomedical Engineering & Instrumentation, NIH

AMHTLC   7
Wesley Hall, M.D.
Past-President, American Medical Association

Health Evaluation: An Entry to the Health Care System   13
Sidney Garfield, M.D.
Founder, Kaiser Foundation Health Plan, Inc.

PLENARY SESSION II

Measurements of Effectiveness of
Health Evaluation Systems   23
Morris F. Collen B.E.E., M.D.
Medical Director, Permanente Medical Group

The People-System   27
Robert E. Westlake, M.D.
Past-President, American Society of
Internal Medicine

Health Evaluation in Transition   33
Anne R. Somers
Rutgers Medical School

PRESIDENTIAL ADDRESS

The Critical Issue: Normal or Normative?   45
Dean F. Davies, M.D., Ph.D.
University of Tennessee School of Medicine

BANQUET ADDRESS

Technology's Role in Health Evaluation   55
John R. Kernodle, M.D.
Chairman, Board of Trustees, AMA

HEALTH EVALUATION IN VARIOUS SETTINGS

AMHT in the Metropolitan Hospital 61
Harry Hochstadt
Executive Vice-President, Cedars of Lebanon
Hospital, Miami, Florida

The Potential Role of AMHT in Evaluation of HMOs 65
Harry E. Emlet, Jr.
Analytic Services, Inc.

Admitting Screening at Latter-Day Saints Hospital 71
T. Allan Pryor, Ph.D. and Homer R. Warner, M.D., Ph.D.
Latter-Day Saints Hospital, Salt Lake City, Utah

An AMHT Program: Its Use in the Care of the Sick and
Evaluation of the Asymptomatic 79
Malcolm Schwartz, M.D.
Automated Screening Centers, Inc.

A Health Testing Concept: Simple-By-Design 83
William R. Duff, Ph.D. and Harry S. Lipscomb, M.D.
Baylor College of Medicine

Entry Point Linkages to
Comprehensive Health Services 89
Melvyn Greberman, M.S., M.D., M.P.H.
U.S. Public Health Service Hospital, Baltimore, Md.

Problems Associated With the
Automated Physician's Assistant 93
Alan H. Purdy, Ph.D.
National Institute for Occupational Safety and Health

Development of the
Automated Physician's Assistant 97
Owen W. Miller, Sc.D., Gayle E. Adams, Ph.D.,
Earl M. Simmons, Jr., M.D. and B. J. Bass, M.D.
University of Missouri Medical Center

The Automated AFEES Project 109
Major Rudolf G. Bickel, USAF, MC
USAF School of Aerospace Medicine

AMHTS and the VA Admission Procedure 115
Richard E. Gordon, M.D., Ph.D., Charles Holzer, B.A.,
Leslie Bielen, M.Ed., Anne Watts, D.A.S.S.
and Katherine L. Gordon
University of Florida College of Medicine

The Role of AMHT in Health Care Systems 125
James L. Craig, M.D.
Director of Medical Services, Tennessee Valley Authority

SPECIAL ASPECTS OF HEALTH EVALUATION
Objective Measurements of
Early Vascular Disease 135
Robert D. Allison, Ph.D.
Scott and White Clinic, Temple, Texas

Coronary Profile: Ethical Considerations 141
William B. Kannel, M.D.
Medical Director, NIH Heart Disease Epidemiology Study

Report Form of the Automated ECG From Considerations
for Acceptability and Efficiency 151
Russell L. Sandberg, M.D.
University of Missouri Medical Center

The Printout as the End Product of AMHT 157
H. A. Haessler, M.D., T. K. Holland
and E. L. Elshtain
Searle Medidata, Inc.

The Pre-Printed Form 159
Emerson Day
Medequip Corporation

Well-Patient Examinations:
Accessibility and Load on Facilities 163
Lawrence I. Schneider
International Health Systems, Inc.

Major Problems in the Early Detection
of Mental Illness 167
Roger Peele, M.D.
St. Elizabeth's Hospital, Washington, D.C.

Value of Biochemical Profiling in a
Periodic Health Examination Program:
Analysis of 1000 Cases 171
W. R. Cunnick, M.D., J. B. Cromie, M.D.,
Ruth Cortell, M.D., Barbara Wright, M.D.,
Eliot Beach, Ph.D., Frederic Seltzer, F.S.A.
and Sybil Miller
Metropolitan Life Insurance Company

CONTENTS (Continued)

Automated Urinalysis: Feasibility and
Clinical Value 189
  DeWitt T. Hunter, Jr., M.D. and Philip A. Fidel, M.S.
  Latter-Day Saints Hospital, Salt Lake City, Utah

Health Data Management: Ontario Plan 197
  Donald J. Shepley, M.D.
  The Hospital for Sick Children, Toronto, Canada

Preface

Up until its Third Annual Scientific Meeting, which this volume reports, the Society for Advanced Medical Systems was a small, under-staffed, poorly supported society. Its seeming weakness, however, was illusory. Its strength lay and continues to abide in a core of dedicated men with a vision to the future.

The first annual meeting, at Deerfield Academy, Deerfield, Massachusetts, was co-sponsored by the Engineering Foundation. The Society's major contribution was the organization of part of the program.

Progress was noted at the Second Annual Scientific Meeting, held at the U.S. Public Health Service Hospital in Baltimore, Maryland. The program included ten papers presented by the staff of the hospital, and the proceedings were printed by the Superintendent of Documents, U.S. Government Printing Office. It was an appropriate first-step for the little society to go-it-alone.

The Third Annual Scientific Meeting was considerably expanded with two plenary and several colloquia sessions, papers being solicited from both members and non-members. The success of the meeting is reflected in the contents of this volume, more timely both here and abroad today than they were when they were presented.

Major papers include six by outstanding leaders in medicine and engineering, the Presidential Address and a Banquet Address. The balance of the meeting had a colloquia format with formal papers and informal presentations. Active exchange of information and views took place in smaller group meetings. For purposes of publication the papers submitted have been grouped in two major categories: Health Evaluation in Various Settings and Special Aspects of Health Evaluation.

Dean F. Davies, M.D., Editor
Past-President, Society for
Advanced Medical Systems

James Tchobanoff, A.M.L.S.
Associate Editor

Acknowledgments

Credit for the success of the meeting and this book can be attributed to all who attended and to those who participated in planning the meeting. Dr. Marshall F. Driggs deserves a special word of appreciation as Program Chairman. Volunteers on the local Arrangements Committee gave generously of their time and included Dr. Bland Cannon, Dr. Glen Clark, Mrs. Pat Vanderschaaf, George Koenig, Wallace Mayton and Jack Aldridge.

Special appreciation must go to Mrs. Marian Frye, who gave above-and-beyond service. Volunteers included Alice Davies, Karen Nelson, Kay Frye, Nancy Davies and Eugenia Derryberry. Work on the manuscripts was fitted into already overloaded schedules by Mrs. Shirley Schultz, Mrs. Linda Montgomery and others on the Editor's staff.

James Tchobanoff, Associate Editor, performed an invaluable editorial service in partial fulfillment of his responsibility in the University of Tennessee Postgraduate Training Program for Science Librarians. The Editor was his preceptor in the Program. Appreciation is extended to Dr. Andrew Lasslo and Mr. Jess Martin for making this arrangement possible.

D.F.D.

Welcoming Address

We welcome you to Memphis and the U.T. Medical Units. It is a pleasure and honor to have you with us. We are honored to have such distinguished participants. We are particularly delighted to have Dr. Wesley Hall, President of the AMA, with us. I am also very proud that Dr. Dean Davies is President of this outstanding organization.

I welcome you, wearing two hats: as a Vice-President of the entire U.T. system and as Chancellor of this campus, the U.T. Medical Units. Our medical units have been one of the largest in the nation. Up until five or six years ago, our enrollment was the largest of any medical complex in the country. We now have the fifth largest medical education complex in the nation. The University of Tennessee is taking in 200 students a year and graduating them 36 months thereafter. In some ways we are not really proud of that because we would really like to be smaller, to be growing and taking advantage of federal funds resulting from growth. Unfortunately, we did our growing back in the 50s when a member of the Tennessee Legislature called for a physician one night for his wife and couldn't get one. At that point in time, by legislative action, our enrollment was increased from about 100 to 200 entering students a year. We have been trying to catch up with that action in terms of facilities and staff ever since. So, currently we are not doing much to increase enrollment, but we are trying to enhance the quality of our educational program.

Among these things, we are establishing some clinical campuses in the eastern part of this state, some 400 miles away. Believe it or not, we have a medical school in Memphis without a University-owned hospital and we have a University-owned hospital in Knoxville, 400 miles away, without a medical school. I have never been quite able to explain how that happened, but it is true.

The University of Tennessee Medical Units has some unique features that cause us to be particularly interested in the theme of this conference. We are proud of the fact that our Chronic Disease Detection Program (now Prevention Clinic) was established some time ago. It was apparently the first multiphasic screening-type program in the country based in a medical school. We are also proud of a relationship between our College of Medicine and our local Health Department, which is training our own particular brand of nurse practitioner; that is, we are taking public health nurses and training these women to take care of patients with chronic diseases under the guidance of physicians.

Joseph E. Johnson, Ed.D.
Vice-President for Development and Administration
Chancellor of the Medical Units
University of Tennessee, Memphis

The Engineer and Advanced Medical Systems

Lester Goodman

The practice of engineering is an action-oriented, pragmatic activity devoted to devising and implementing methods and apparatus to meet the needs of society. Its armamentarium includes the general body of scientific knowledge, the rational language of mathematics, and a rich background of experience in transforming energy and materials into utilitarian constructs.

In recent years it has been repeatedly and dramatically demonstrated that engineers have much to contribute to biomedical research and health care. Engineer-life scientist and engineer-medical practitioner teams have functioned with a combined productivity far in excess of the sum of individual efforts. Significant portions of the scientific body of knowledge, related to living processes, have been translated and extended by and for engineers. A substantial academic base now exists in the scores of explicit individual and collaborative programs in our universities. Numerous exotic instruments have been developed with which one can detect, measure, process and display biomedical data with unprecedented scope and clarity.

The field called "Biomedical Engineering" has emerged and the cadre of professionals who claim to be "biomedical engineers" numbers in the thousands and continues to grow. Biomedical engineering can be characterized as the *application* of the methodology and technology of the physical sciences and engineering to *problems* in the context of the living system, with emphasis on the diagnosis, treatment and prevention of disorder in man.

As professionals, we are actively concerned with issues of personal and community well being. People are aware that only a small fraction receive adequate health care. Costs of medical services are escalating beyond reach of all but the affluent. These conditions have resulted in massive demands for *application* of science and technology to the immediate alleviation of the multitude of *problems* involved in providing improved health for our entire population. Traditionally, the direct responsibility and authority for

Lester Goodman, Ph.D., *Chief, Biomedical Engineering and Instrumentation Branch, Division of Research Services, National Institutes of Health, Bethesda, Maryland and Past-President, Alliance for Engineering in Medicine and Biology, Washington, D.C.*

1

medical research and patient care has been vested in the life scientist and medical practitioner. This is altogether fitting and proper. We recognize that care of the community is not the unique domain of the medical profession alone; society is best served by the synergism of all pertinent knowledge and skills.

Implicit in this statement is the recognition that neither the engineer nor the man of medicine can contribute effectively in isolation from other disciplines. In almost every case he must function as a member of an appropriate team of specialists. This by no means implies that the engineer, or his counterpart from medicine, is an expert in all pertinent disciplines. It does imply, however, that he is an expert in his field who is willing to learn to communicate with, understand, and respect serious workers from other fields.

The life science researcher or clinical practitioner daily faces problems of measurement, analysis and synthesis that are characterized by a degree of complexity and subtlety far in excess of those encountered in typical engineering and engineered systems. He recognizes the rapid development of new techniques and devices recently developed by the engineer. He senses that these should be of great help to him, but he is often mystified, even baffled, as to how to take advantage of these new resources. He resents, justifiably, the intrusion and criticism of the glib engineer with his "exact" physical laws, "exact" mathematics and "exact" electronic computers. The engineer, on the other hand, senses that he has much to offer biology and medicine. He, too, justifiably resents the traditions and empiricism of much of medical practice and research and its reluctance to accept what modern technology can provide. Too often, the natural boundary that exists between the life and the physical sciences has developed into a formidable barrier because of naive dilettantism and arrogance on both sides. These barriers can be avoided and those that do exist can be broken down if, and only if, free exchange of ideas and mutual respect are enhanced.

The often cited "communications gap" closes rapidly when competent workers from several disciplines meet together with an individual and collective motivation to define and solve problems rather than to protect personal prerogatives, traditional authority and prestige, dogmatic shibboleths and the pocketbook.

It would serve little purpose here to cite and illustrate examples where engineer and medical teamwork has provided significant contributions to health care and humanity. Laboratories and clinics are well equipped with instruments and systems designed and built by engineers with the guidance of life scientists and medical practitioners. Professional journals and the popular press are replete with articles and advertisements describing new techniques and apparatus.

This discussion will offer comment upon a recent development of widespread relevance in the field. It, too, is an example of teamwork by people from many disciplines concerned with the nation's health. In this case the purpose is to seek effective mechanisms whereby workers from disparate specialties can communicate and work together, with an individual and collective motivation to share knowledge, experience and resources in a mutual effort to improve health care for all.

This is a system that is yet in an early development stage, barely two years off the drawing board; one that has been designed upon many years of experience and, it is hoped, will perform more effectively than earlier prototypes. It is called the Alliance for Engineering in Medicine and Biology (AEMB). The Society for Advanced Medical Systems is an important structural and active element of the Alliance.

To trace the complete genealogy of the AEMB is far too complex a task, there now being 20 members of the family, each of which is a professional association of national scope and each of which has its own family tree. For sake of perspective, it may be informative briefly to describe a main trunk.

In 1948, in New York City, a group of engineers from the Instrument Society of America (ISA) and the American Institute of Electrical Engineers (AIEE), with professional interests in the areas of x-ray and radiation apparatus used in medicine, held the First Annual Conference on Medical Electronics. Soon thereafter the Institute of Radio Engineers (IRE) joined with the ISA and the AIEE and the series of annual meetings continued. Subsequent years witnessed a remarkable growth of interest in biomedical engineering and participation by other technical associations. By 1968 the original core group evolved into the Joint Committee on Engineering in Medicine and Biology (JCEMB) with five adherent national society members: the Instrument Society of America (ISA), the Institute of Electrical and Electronics Engineers, Inc. (IEEE), the American Society of Mechanical Engineers (ASME), the American Institute of Chemical Engineers (AIChE), and the Association for the Advancement of Medical Instrumentation (AAMI), who jointly conducted the annual conference which had been renamed the Annual Conference on Engineering in Medicine and Biology (ACEMB).

Professional groups responded vigorously to the demands of the times. Attendance at the annual conference by natural scientists and medical practitioners grew to approximately 40% of the total; medical associations were requesting formal participation with their technical counterparts on the JCEMB. New interdisciplinary organizations were formed. New intrasociety and intersociety groups, committees, councils, etc., became active. Resources were readily available in the 1960s; meetings filled the calendar and publications overflowed the shelves. Unfortunately, in too

many cases, individual competitions for positions of leadership and
authority displaced motivations to develop the coordinated program of
efforts required to best serve the professions and the community.

In 1968 a document was prepared that read:

SALIENT ISSUES

Whereas:
1. Common interdisciplinary purposes cannot be well served by individual groups working independently from each other;
2. Certain associations have developed in attempts to meet the need;
3. Conferences and publications have proliferated in attempts to meet
   the need;
4. At present, no mutually satisfactory mechanism exists for the
   coordination of the relevant groups and functions;
5. There does exist an annual meeting and proceedings publication
   sponsored by a limited number of societies through the Joint
   Committee on Engineering in Medicine and Biology (JCEMB);
6. The JCEMB is formally structured with a constitution, plural societal
   representation, and an established pattern of operation. This structure and pattern of operation, however, are not deemed adequate to
   fulfill present and future needs. To the best of our knowledge, there
   exists no other single organization that seems capable of fulfilling
   these needs.
Therefore, it is appropriate that a new organization be established.

On July 21, 1969, at the 22nd ACEMB in Chicago, Illinois,
representatives of 14 national engineering, scientific and medical associations founded the Alliance for Engineering in Medicine and Biology
(AEMB). As of today, the AEMB consists of 20 such organizations; its
operations are determined by an Administrative Council composed of
delegates from each of its affiliates.

These include: the Aerospace Medical Association, the American
Academy of Orthopaedic Surgeons, the American Association of Physi-
cists in Medicine, the American College of Physicians, the American
College of Radiology, the American College of Surgeons, the American
Institute for Ultrasonics in Medicine, the American Institute of Biologi-
cal Sciences, the American Institute of Chemical Engineers, the Ameri-
can Society for Engineering Education, the American Society for Testing
and Materials, the American Society for Heating, Refrigeration and
Air-Conditioning Engineers, Inc., the American Society for Internal
Medicine, the American Society of Agricultural Engineers, the American
Society of Mechanical Engineers, the Association for the Advancement
of Medical Instrumentation, the Institute of Electrical and Electronics
Engineers, Inc., the Instrument Society of America, the Neuroelectric
Society, and the Society for Advanced Medical Systems.

The essential character of the Alliance can be conveyed by excerpts from its constitution, bylaws, and recorded minutes:

To promote cooperation among associations which have an active interest in the interaction of engineering and the physical sciences with medicine and the biological sciences in enhancement of biomedical knowledge and health care.

The AEMB shall assume no jurisdiction in connection with the proprietary activities or policies of constituent associations.

... to establish an environment and mechanisms whereby people from relevant various disciplines can be motivated and stimulated to work together . . .

... respond to the needs of its member societies, as expressed by their delegates, rather than to seek authoritative preeminence in its domain of interest . . .

... support and enhance the professional activities of its membership . . .

The AEMB is now just two years old. Efforts, to date, have been devoted primarily to establishing working relationships among its members, structural and functional mechanisms for conducting its affairs and fulfilling responsibilities inherited from its predecessor, the JCEMB. The 23rd ACEMB, the first under the aegis of the Alliance, was held in Washington, D. C., in November 1970. Planning and preliminary implementation actions are underway for conferences through 1975.

The Alliance is assured of an active role on the world scene by virtue of its formal affiliation with the International Federation for Medical and Biological Engineering (IFMBE). The AEMB was represented at the meetings of the IFMBE General Assembly held August 1970 in Melbourne, Australia, at the 9th International Conference on Medical and Biological Engineering. The 10th International Conference is scheduled for August 1973 in Dresden, German Democratic Republic.

In conclusion, we have a very rich medical science and a powerful technology. There are no permanent technical impasses to the solution of biomedical problems. Simply put, if together we can define a problem and together apply our individual and collective knowledge and skills, then together we can find the solutions we seek.

AMHTLC

Wesley Hall

I would like to discuss the subject of AMHTLC. I have not joined the ranks of those in Federal Service who are fascinated by strings of initials from which to hang various agencies and I am not going to talk in some kind of code, but I am going to talk about a code, a particular code. As to the title of this address, "AMHTLC," we all know that AMHT stands for Automated Multiphasic Health Testing. I add the LC for a little play on words, also utilizing the preceding letter T, giving us TLC. We know that usually stands for Tender Loving Care. In the medical and health professions, tender loving care is known under various other names: concern, patience, understanding, kindness — all those words are a part of a code, a code originated in the days of Galen and Hippocrates and followed to this day by all good physicians, the code of caring for the patient. Such a code is particularly meaningful to multiphasic testing operations. They represent a tremendous advance in the health field and I commend the technical skills and the enterprise which lay behind that advance. However, the field of multiphasic testing is not without its hurdles and possible pitfalls. Not the least of the hurdles is acceptance of AMHT by the public and the medical profession.

This is a curious country. Americans are known for eagerly accepting the new, the progressive, the better way, the efficient way, but sometimes there is a paradox. Americans applaud the innovative and efficient but often deplore anything smacking of the assembly line, automated operation. Many today now denounce such operations as depersonalizing and dehumanizing. Possibly they might be, but they need not be. Those involved with AMHT must be especially careful in this regard. It is not merely a question of gearing up our health services to run large numbers of people through various tests and evaluations. A very important consideration is how they are run through. It must never become a push-pull, click-click type of thing, with the patient viewed much as a carton to be packed at various stations along an assembly line. It must never be set up as something independent of the medical doctor — a sort of do-it-yourself quick physical check-up kit — and it must always be operated under the

Wesley Hall, M.D., *Past-President, American Medical Association, Chicago, Ill.*

concept of being an important part of the total health team picture. We have seen some disturbing things and the American Medical Association has expressed its concern. A recent statement of AMA's judicial council addresses itself to the multiphasic testing and makes several points.

First of all, let it be said that AMHT offers a very useful extension of health services under certain guidelines. Primary among them is that AMHT is a fact-finding and reporting system. Findings disclosed by such tests should be interpreted only by physicians for patients. Multiphasic testing is not a diagnosis. All AMHTs should be closely linked and coordinated with the local medical society, hospitals, medical centers and doctors. This is to the benefit of all concerned.

It is obvious that there will be confusion on the part of the patients as to the true function of AMHT. Many will see it as a mysterious, space age, computer doctor who lacks only the old manufacturing slogan, "untouched by human hands." Unfortunately, as our Judicial Council points out, some testing facilities have given the appearance, at least, of encouraging individuals to be tested without a medical referral for the test. Some appear to be operated without any communication with the attending physician. Some perform a battery of tests, none of which were requested by the attending physician. To quote from the council statement: "No ethical physician would wish to be associated with such a plan because it fails to consider sound medical advice in providing health care at a cost commensurate with the services rendered." Such examples are, of course, a definite minority. Most testing facilities strive to be, and are, high-quality components of our health care system. A guard must be up at times — and I am not singling out AMHT when I emphasize close connection with the medical profession. The AMA feels the same way about blood banks, for example. It urges that a physician exercise constant supervision and that blood bank activities be coordinated with local medical societies and hospitals. You know the problem that we have had with blood banks and their commercialization. The point of it all is that whether dealing with blood, vital human tissue or with other aspects of health care, such as multiphasic health testing, one must never lose sight of the sense of dedication, of attention to quality, and of concern which is embodied in the code, because you are dealing with people. If you make it plain to patients and physicians that AMHT can provide real benefits within a context of total medical service performed with a genuine feeling for the patients, then you have the basic foundation for acceptance. Some say that many doctors are reluctant to accept AMHT out of fear of being displaced, or of losing control of the practice of medicine, or of becoming a mere technician. That, I submit, is not the case. You know the limits of AMHT better than I. There is not and never will be a truly automated diagnosis. The physician is still indispensable.

Some doctors shy away from the term "computers in medicine" but the AMA has a vigorous program of studying, evaluating and planning in regard to computers. Computers represent a useful tool just as a better designed scalpel or retractor represents a more useful tool for the surgeons. Someday computers will help a doctor make a diagnosis providing him in minutes, endless information that would take him weeks to dig out in a medical library. That can save thousands of lives, so we want such a development just as fast as we can get it. This is the position of the American Medical Association.

Doctors are not dinosaurs, despite what some critics might say. If they were, they would never adopt anything new, and instead of implanting heart valves under the skin and in the heart, we would be putting leeches on the skin and not be concerned with the real problem of defective heart valves. History of medical progress has been a history of recognizing, carefully testing and then adopting new tools, techniques, drugs, or methods which would clearly help physicians do their job. It is apparent that AMHT can be of inestimable help. Doctors must be convinced of the soundness of any new procedure. Sometimes doctors are a little hard to convince of the things that are new, and, unfortunately, some members of our profession refuse to advance with the advancements of the times. New procedures and systems must be sold on the basis of respect for the physician and his proper place, on dedication to a well-planned and well-run operation, and with due overall concern for the benefit of the patient. It is not the best procedure to take people in off the street, test them and send the results to a physician whose name the test subject took out of a telephone book. That is haphazard health care. Follow-up should be carefully planned. One cannot look at it as what is new or what is old in the context of simple entities. One must look at the total picture. Dr. Edward Annis, former AMA president, said something recently which might be applied here. We must remember doctors should never be reduced to technician status, but should remain a highly respected, indeed a revered figure, as he has been since antiquity, because of his extensive training and knowledge. The ultimate success or failure of our industry as a private industry lies not in the kind of care we can provide but in the efficiency with which we make it available equally to all people of this nation, in the compassion with which we apply it to the individual patient and the ease with which each patient can avail himself of our services. These are the key factors: efficiency such as is represented by AMHT and compassion in applying that efficiency.

Now how do you sell doctors on the AMHT? By working with them, by communicating with them, by cooperating in the total health effort for patients' benefit. Show physicians this kind of spirit and demonstrate a capacity for providing reliable data. In at least one case, an AMHT center really put doctors to the test very successfully. In Kings County, New York, 210 doctors were invited to undergo multiphasic testing and 206 of them showed up — a fine batting average for doctors. Reportedly, 73% of the group believed such tests were appropriate before the examinations were given; afterwards, 92% of them felt that they were very appropriate and rewarding. This is in the medical profession — 92%. This is what I call education. AMHT should be truly integrated into community health systems. Who is in a better position to advise on such matters as expected patient volume as the doctors or the medical society? How better can planning and activities be guided through knowledge of the needs? There is much AMHT can contribute. Not the least is the providing of comprehensive health testing at a much lower cost than that prevailing under older methods. Pre-hospital admission testing is a great service. As for helping the physician, let me cite the experience at a multiphasic testing center near Chicago. In six months, three internists performed twice as many comprehensive adult examinations as they had been able to perform the same period of time the previous year. Waiting time for examinations was reduced from three months to two weeks. My, what an answer to our critics in helping settle our health problem with regard to the supply of medical care in all facets!

There is a shortage of physicians in some areas. There is a super-saturation of physicians in other areas. Despite many valiant efforts to correct this situation, such as the opening of a record number of medical schools, it still takes time to train a doctor — a lot of time. The duties and responsibilities of a physician demand careful preparation. Anything that can make the physicians we have more effective is thus important. Now actually in regard to AMHT, we stand at a point very early in the game: various bugs have to be worked out and techniques and procedures need to be refined. One area is the printout of test results; they must counsel, not confuse. Once the moving machine has done its work, the doctor should be able to read what is written. But that and other problems, I am confident, will be solved. I am also confident that more and more physicians will come to accept multiphasic screening as a useful tool. Acceptance of anything usually takes some time. After all, at the dawn of time, God breathed life into man, but it took the American Red Cross until 1951 to come out with mouth-to-mouth resuscitation.

I hope that I have conveyed a basic idea that cooperation, mutual respect-understanding usually result in concrete achievement. Multiphasic health testing holds great promise and potential as a new phase of health care and it could not offer that unless good people were involved in it. I have no doubt at all that our joint efforts will truly mesh into a much stronger, much better health care system. AMHT might well stand for Allies in Medical Health Technology — all who are involved in trying to

keep people well or make them well are allies. It is a big job. We need all
the help we can get. Those who have devoted so many years to perfecting
the type of technology that is going to be indispensable for the medical
profession in the near future are to be commended for their efforts and
their work. Now let us all join hand in hand in developing, in perfecting as
nearly as possible, and in utilizing every adjunct to the overall challenge of
providing quality health care for all Americans at the most reasonable cost
possible.

Health Evaluation:
An Entry to the Health Care System

Sidney Garfield

U. S. medicine is in serious trouble. Shortages of manpower, unavailability of services and runaway costs are creating tremendous pressures for legislation, most of which focuses on national health insurance and prepaid group practice patterned after Kaiser-Permanente as a solution.

National health insurance will only make matters worse. The present medical crisis was precipitated by Medicare and Medicaid and the surge of demand they produced. It is sheer folly to believe that compounding that demand by expanding health insurance to the entire population will improve matters — on the contrary, further overtaxing the faltering delivery system will certainly deteriorate the quality and availability of care for the sick.

As for prepaid group practice — though it is flattering to have part of our program proposed as a model for this nation's future delivery system — it is a mistake to believe that it will automatically solve very much. There is nothing inherent in prepaid group practice that guarantees ready availability of service. In fact, this has been as serious a problem with us as in practice in general. Prepayment makes medical care a right by eliminating fee-for-service, and for years we have been deeply concerned with our relative ability to keep up with the soaring demand that this right produces and to maintain a satisfactory level of service.

Striving to solve this problem and improve our services, we have uncovered a basic defect in the delivery system that has somehow passed unnoticed by us and the rest of the medical world. Recognizing this defect and its cause is extremely important since its correction is the key to solving most of this nation's medical care problems and leads to a great opportunity for all of us.

Let us first consider the traditional medical care delivery system (Fig. 1). Customarily, the patient decides when he needs care. This more or less educated decision by the patient creates a variable mix input composed of well, "worried well," "early sick" and sick people. In traditional practice

Sidney Garfield, M.D., *Founder, Kaiser Foundation Health Plan, Inc., Oakland, Calif.*

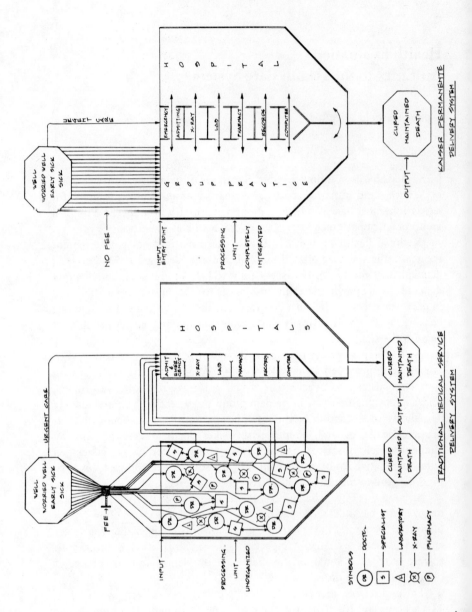

Figure 1.

the patient enters knowing he is to pay a fee. The processing unit consists of individual discrete medical care resources (doctors, labs, x-rays, hospitals, etc.). The output is a cured patient — hopefully.

The Kaiser-Permanente program alters that traditional medical care delivery system in just two ways. It eliminates the fee for service, substituting prepayment, and it structures the discrete units of medical care resources into a well-organized group practice in integrated clinic and hospital facilities. Much of the economic advantage of our Plan derives from this organization. However, it should be pointed out this does not arise from group practice per se, but rather from the total integration of doctors, clinics, hospitals and ancillary services.

The defect we have uncovered is related to the elimination of fee. The obvious purpose of the fee is to remunerate the doctor. It has a less obvious but important side effect: it is a potent regulator of flow into the delivery system. Since nobody wants to pay for unneeded medical care, there is a tendency to put off seeing the doctor until one is really sick. This limits the number of people seeking entry, particularly the well and early sick. Conversely, the sicker a person is, the earlier he seeks help — regardless of fee. Thus, the fee-for-service regulator (Fig. 2) limits quantity, minimizes the well and early sick and maximizes the sick in the entry mix. With the input of fee-for-service predominantly sick people, the system that has evolved over the years to match that input is a sick-care delivery system, with the doctor at the point of entry and deeply involved in every step of the sick-care process. Likewise, our medical schools have evolved concentrating on teaching sick-care technology.

Elimination of the fee has always been a primary objective of our Plan since it acts as a barrier to early entry into sick care. Early entry is essential for early treatment and prevention of serious illness and complications. It is distressing to realize that elimination of fees can be as much of a barrier to early care as the fee itself. The reason is that when we removed the fee, we removed that regulator of flow into the system. The result is a massive, uncontrolled flood of the entire variable mix, the well, the worried well, the early sick and the sick, into the point of entry — the doctor's appointment — on a first-come, first-served basis that has little relation to priority of need. The impact of this demand overloads the system and, since the well and worried well are a large component of that entry mix, their usurping of doctor time actually acts as a barrier to entry of the sick.

This same thing is happening to medical care throughout the country. The traditional delivery system, which has evolved under fee for service, is being overwhelmed because of the elimination of personally paid fees through the spread of health insurance, Medicare and Medicaid. This floods the system not only with increased numbers of people but with that

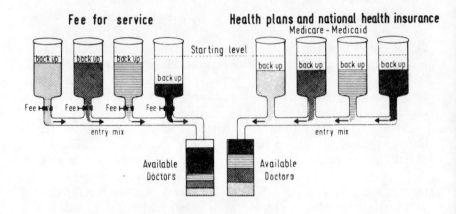

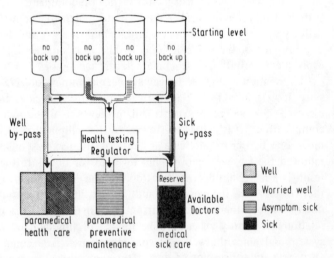

Figure 2.

same altered entry mix containing a large proportion of relatively well people. For this considerable segment of patients, the old methods of work-up by the physician become very inefficient. He spends a large portion of his time trying to find something wrong with well people, using techniques he was taught for diagnosing illness. This reverse use of sick-care technology, searching for illness in healthy people, is extremely wasteful of doctor's time, and in addition, is boring and frustrating for him.

This is the defect we have uncovered. The altered entry mix created by the elimination of personally paid fees, as occurs in health plans, Medicare, Medicaid and medical care as a right, is incompatible with direct entry into today's sick-care delivery system. It is incompatible because the mismatch it creates drastically dissipates and wastes medical manpower.

Correcting this defect requires a new system design that realistically matches the altered entry mix of free care. This necessitates two things: first, a regulator of flow into the system that can separate the variable mix into its three basic components — the well, the asymptomatic sick and the sick; and second, an adequate service to receive each of those components. The regulator we have developed is "Health Testing." The services are a new "Health-Care Service" for the well, a new "Preventive-Maintenance Service" for the asymptomatic sick, and a pure "Sick-Care Service" for the sick.

The new system thus has four divisions (Fig. 3):

1. *Multiphasic Health Testing* — the heart of the new system — combines a detailed automated medical history with comprehensive panels of physiological and laboratory tests administered by paramedical personnel. Originally designed in our operations to meet the ever-increasing demand for health checkups, health testing is ideally suited as a new method of entry into medical care since it can effectively separate the entry mix into its components with a minimum of physician involvement.

2. *Health Care* is a new division of medicine that does not exist in this country or any country. Its purpose is to improve health and keep people well. To date, health care has been an elusive concept, and understandably so, since it has been submerged in sick care — the primary concern of doctors. Doctors trained in sick care have been much too busy to be involved with well people.

   This clear definition of a Health-Care Service is a first step in creating a positive program for keeping people well. Whether or not one believes this can be done is beside the point. This service is essential to meet the increasing demand for health care and to keep these people from using up sick-care services.

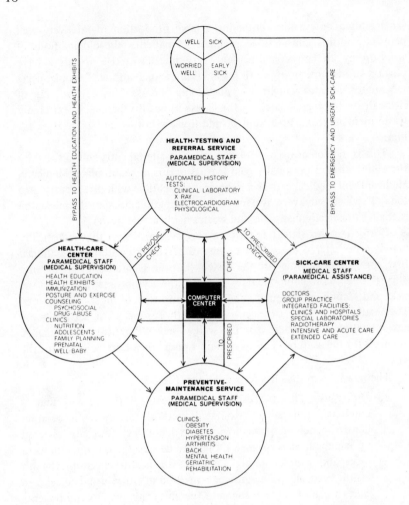

Figure 3.

3. *Preventive Maintenance* is a service for the asymptomatic sick and high-prevalence chronic illnesses, such as hypertension and diabetes, that require monitoring and surveillance. This type of care performed by paramedical personnel reporting to the patient's doctor can relieve the physician of many routine visits.

4. *Sick Care*, with its high-level decisions on diagnosis and therapy, becomes clearly the realm of the physician. Here he becomes the manager of patient care rather than the man of all work and is aided in this by all three of the other divisions.

There are several important features to be emphasized in this new delivery system:

1. It is designed specifically to match the entry mix of free care. All other existing systems, including Great Britain's, unload the entire free-care entry mix into sick care and thus dissipate and waste medical manpower.

2. Three of the four divisions — Health Testing, Health Care and Preventive Maintenance — are primarily automated and paramedical services of existing types. Therefore, they are relatively easy to staff and relatively inexpensive. The use of paramedical personnel with limited knowledge and skills to relieve the physician of routine and repetitious tasks requires such tasks be clearly defined and structured. The existing delivery system with its unstructured heterogeneous entry mix is almost the exact antithesis of those requirements and, therefore, has never permitted effective and safe use of such personnel. For this reason Health Testing and the clear separation of services, automatically defining tasks and structure, become the key to paramedical manpower effectiveness.

3. This new system requires no restructuring of sick-care services. It can function with either solo practice or group practice. All we need do to sick care is remove from it the extraneous portion of the entry mix produced by free care, which did not belong there in the first place. Sick care relieved of that considerable load of well, worried well and asymptomatic sick people thus develops a greatly increased capacity for the care of the sick.

4. Past medical care has been crisis-oriented and episodic with the patient entering when he believed he was ill and leaving the system when pronounced cured. This new system permits a fresh approach to that process. Health Testing and the conditions it reveals make it possible to plan not only the immediate services needed by the patient but also to schedule returns for updating the health profile from that point. Thus the system can now tell the patient when to enter for care. Today all new entries into medical care are potential emergencies since we have no foresight of the patient's condition; under this new system only visits between scheduled returns for updating are emergencies. The medical reason for these unscheduled visits can then be diagnosed against a background of health profile rechecks — all rapidly retrievable by computer techniques. In this fashion a large segment of medical care can be continuous rather than episodic, much of illness a trend rather than a crisis, and treatment preventive rather than "putting out fires." This is the type of system that best fits medical care as a right.

It should be clear that the cause of today's medical care crisis has been the inexorable spread of free care throughout our population. The effect is an expanded and altered demand that is incompatible with the existing sick care-delivery system, wasting its medical manpower and threatening the quality and economics of the service it renders.

It is grossly unfair to blame that effect on the medical profession. The delivery system functioned fairly well with fee-for-service under which it evolved. It became unbalanced and a so-called non-system under the impact of the poorly planned legislation of Medicare and Medicaid with its elimination of fees, and that result should not surprise anyone. Picture what would happen to air transportation if fares were eliminated and travel became a right. What chance would you have getting anyplace if you really needed to? Even the highly automated telephone service would be staggered by removal of fees and necessary calls would become practically impossible. The change from "fee" to "free" would disrupt any system in the country, no matter how well organized, and this is particularly true of medicine with its highly personalized sick-care service.

Nevertheless, legislation is on the move and if we are to have more free care — and it appears we will — it is crucial this time that a rational delivery system be prepared for the inevitable deluge of demand, so that we can preserve the basic medical values we believe in. These values include quality of care, availability of service and reasonable economics. Morally and practically, they should also include the freedom to practice individually, or in groups, as best suits the needs of the people to be served and the physicians who serve them.

Prodding physicians against their desires into group practice will result in less production and less service, not more. Prepaid group practice requires an unusual dedication to that form of service and that dedication is relatively scarce and cannot be dictated or legislated. Actually, at this point in time, we need both types of practice. It is most important that we preserve freedom of choice and changes should be evolutionary, not forced.

Viewed from our long experience with medical care as a right, the organization of practice is not the issue anyway. Neither solo practice nor group practice will function efficiently and without great waste of medical manpower until the delivery system matches the altered input of free care. This requires the missing services of Health Testing, Health Care and Preventive Maintenance. Without them the demand of free care can only deteriorate services for all and quality care as a right becomes impossible.

As for the major legislative proposals to date, these seem to be strangely paradoxical. They would exponentially increase demand and at the same time, through mistaken emphasis on forcing group practice, might decrease productivity. They would massively flood the delivery system by eliminating fees and at the same time destroy incentives to serve by capitation, salaries and limiting budgets. They would force an unconscionable load of well and sick on the medical profession and at the same time destroy their morale by taking away their freedom of choice on their methods of practice. A truly questionable design for the future delivery system and certainly one that is unlikely to preserve our medical values.

If there is validity in these arguments, American Medicine should back medical care as a right, with the provision that it be carefully planned to preserve basic medical values. This means advocating a two- to three-year period of preparation during which those essential paramedical services would be established throughout the country, prior to making free care effective. Hopefully, this would be done by our medical societies, with financing by some such mechanism as the $800 million Resource Development Fund being proposed to stimulate group practice. A similar fund to establish these paramedical services would be extremely effective in bringing direct early improvement to medical services for the people.

Medical care stands at a critical point. One path is legislation that, with minor variations, compounds the errors of Medicare and Medicaid and can only depreciate the quality and availability of care for both the sick and well. The better route is to create a new delivery system that recognizes free care is not just sick care but encompasses the entire spectrum of health — a system that by matching that spectrum will make it genuinely possible to achieve the principle of quality medical care as a right and preserve the best of our present medical values. That choice is our opportunity.

This paper was originally entitled, "Prevention of dissipation of health services resources," published in the *American Journal of Public Health* 61:1499-1506 (August 1971), and is reprinted by permission.

Measurements of Effectiveness of Health Evaluation Systems

Morris F. Collen

Introduction

The development of large technological systems requires large investments of capital over long periods of time. As a result, it is essential to carefully evaluate the effectiveness of such systems in achieving their defined health care objectives and their efficiency in the use of costly resources.

In measuring the efficiency of a physical system, the engineer defines efficiency as the ratio of output to input. In health care systems, the evaluation of program efficiency has similarly been defined by Deniston[1] as the ratio between an output (new attainment of program objectives), and an input (program resources expended, usually expressed as average dollar costs). Often this ratio is inverted and expressed, for example, as dollar cost per positive case for multiphasic screening.[2] The measurement of the degree of attainment of program objectives is usually defined as the effectiveness of the program. Program effectiveness is thus the ratio of the attained objectives attributed to the program activity to the proposed objectives to be attained by the program activity.[3]

Quantifiable measures of all relevant inputs and outputs to health care systems are usually impossible to obtain. Thorner[4] has suggested that determinations of incremental changes in health (as program objectives or outputs) and in health services (as inputs) are the usual measures applied to evaluation of health care programs. Flagle[5] has described a model to develop evaluation criteria which, for example, in a medical information system include volume and completeness; timeliness and process speed; reliability and accuracy; operability, utility and acceptability; and cost. These criteria have been applied by Richart,[6] utilizing comparison measurements to both baseline conditions and to other similar control systems. Thus, in measuring the efficiency of a health care system, or a subsystem, one must (1) carefully and explicitly define appropriate

Morris F. Collen, B.E.E., M.D., *Director, Medical Methods Research, Permanente Medical Group, Oakland, Calif.; President, Society for Advanced Medical Systems.*

attainable objectives for a defined time period, such as immediate and/or long term; (2) define criteria for evaluation of effectiveness of program, i.e., measures of degree of attainment of the defined objectives and of the resources expended in the specified times; and (3) collect measurements of these outputs and inputs through time, so as to permit determinations of incremental changes as compared to some reasonably valid controls.

Effectiveness of a Multiphasic
Health Testing System

The assessment of the effectiveness of multiphasic health testing for periodic health examinations is an example of a health care subsystem evaluation. Two alternative methods for providing periodic health examinations are available: the traditional method and the multiphasic health checkup.

The objectives of multiphasic testing are defined as follows:
1. Effective health surveillance and disease detection
2. Effective monitoring of chronic disease and treatment
3. Achievement of high level patient acceptability
4. Improved quality of testing
5. Conservation of physician time
6. Improved service to patients
7. Decreased costs of health testing
8. Decreases in disability, morbidity and mortality.

The effectiveness of the multiphasic health checkup in achieving objectives 1 through 7 can all be measured within 12-24 months. Objective 8 measures patients' outcome and requires a long-term controlled study.

Effectiveness of a New
Entry System to Medical Care

Another example of the magnitude of effort to evaluate large medical systems is that in progress to test the use of a multiphasic health testing unit as a new entry mode to a medical care delivery system.

The objectives of this project are the following:
1. To utilize a multiphasic Health Testing Service to direct patients to appropriate Health Care, Preventive Care, and Sick Care Services;
2. To utilize paramedical personnel wherever possible, in order to conserve physician time; and
3. To measure the impact of the new system upon conservation of physician time, staff response, patient satisfaction and costs of the new system as compared to the current system for providing medical services.

Conclusion

The determination of the effectiveness of health care systems is time-consuming, difficult and costly. It is essential, however, to conduct properly planned program evaluations if we are to improve efficiency of our health care systems.

References

1. Deniston, O. L., Rosenstock, I. M., Welch, W. et al.: Evaluation of program efficiency. *Pub. Health Rep.*, 83:603-610, 1968.
2. Collen, M. F., Feldman, R., Siegelaub, A. B. et al.: Dollar cost per positive test for automated multiphasic screening. *New. Eng. J. Med.*, 283:459-463, 1970.
3. Deniston, O. L., Rosenstock, I. M. and Getting, V. A.: Evaluation of program effectiveness. *Pub. Health Rep.*, 83:323-335, 1968.
4. Thorner, R. M.: Health program evaluation in relation to health programming. *HSMHA Tech. Health Rep.*, 86:525-532, 1971.
5. Flagle, C. D.: Evaluation techniques for medical information systems. *Comp. Biomed. Res.*, 3:407-414, 1970.
6. Richart, R. H.: Evaluation of a medical data system. *Comp. Biomed. Res.*, 3:415-425, 1970.

The People-System

Robert E. Westlake

Health care in this country has been called everything from a non-system to a disaster. Even those who believe the care available is the best in the world know that its availability is spotty, its quality uneven and its cost uncontrolled.

We all recognize that the best system of facilities and personnel, even when well financed, is of no use to a patient who will not or can not find the way to use it. The behavioral scientist says get them in, no matter what their understanding or choice; the educational psychologist says show it to them and allow them to enter or not. But those of us who call ourselves clinicians, bedside professionals who care for individual patients, say to all concerned: "Give us the chance to care for our patients, individually, competently, appropriately — and don't tell us we have failed as managers, systems analysts, cost accountants, engineers, or sociologists." Clinicians need a system in which they can do their thing comfortably and effectively.

Health care is, therefore, a social art using the tools of science, following society's demands for quality and quantity. The people involved in health care have a dual responsibility. They must educate all the public, from patient to politician, about good health practices, i.e., hygiene. And they must keep themselves well equipped with up-to-date, sharp tools.

Clinicians, whose greatest pleasure is patient care, and who should be doing what they do best, have turned amateur social scientists, actuaries, engineers and even politicians because we need a people-system in medicine.

Since the undercared-for are not necessarily the underdoctored, an extension of the people-system by more doctors will not do. The creation of a secondary, if not second class, people-system of care will also not satisfy the needs for improved health. Only an evolutionary improvement — or if you believe there is no system, creation — of a system for all will suffice.

Robert E. Westlake, M.D., *Past-President, American Society of Internal Medicine, Syracuse, N.Y.*

Public health is the sum of individual health, not statistical data about volume, mortality, normal values or even needs. The people-system must be built about the function and subfunctions involved in individual care, not mass care. Since I have practiced and taught personal care as a specialist for 20 years, as well as consulting and administrating a hospital, leading a Blue Shield board and working in organized medicine, I will presume to describe the functions involved in personal health care. This may lead to useful ideas about an advanced people-system.

The goal of the system is the longest, most comfortable, and depending on one's philosophy, the most productive or most pleasurable life possible. The material we work with is the human organism: body, mind and spirit. In addition to historical and physical data about his body, his mental state and his chemistry, we need to know his habits, his family history and his environment. These data, fed into the prepared — or "programmed" — medical mind, hopefully get sorted out, clustered logically and lead to useful conclusions.

These conclusions in good personal preventive care are, first, the identification of health hazards. In the presence of acute or chronic complaints, the conclusions are diagnoses.

Further investigation of these data with knowledge about possible treatment produces a therapeutic plan.

One, therefore, collects data, checks data, evaluates data, selects data and integrates data for one central function. Information about an individual patient must interact with a background of principles and concepts in someone's mind to produce a diagnostic model. Then a treatment model must be constructed. Both models must be evaluated continuously and modified as needed.

Now, who are the people in this system? Now and in the future, it is useful to divide health professionals into clinical professionals, technical professionals and support professionals.

The clinical professionals are applied scientists in contact with the individual patient. They are concerned with the human being. They are responsible for building the models of diagnoses and treatment. They use data about an individual patient, applying cognitive and affective input, and postulate health hazards, diagnoses and prognoses. They also construct a treatment model and either supervise or implement its operation.

Obviously, the original clinical professional was, and still is, the practicing physician. The need for help in running the treatment model produced nurses.

The physician classically collects his data, diagnoses, then treats. The complexities of *health science* produced technical specialists, either from physicians, or *de novo*. The complexities of *society* produced support professionals, such as social workers, administrators and others.

The modern MD has generally been educated and trained by older MDs to replicate themselves. Doing his own history, examining the patient himself, checking the urine or blood smear — all these are regarded as the mark of a fine clinician. Inductive or deductive reasoning from minimal data, leading to an unusual diagnosis, is regarded as genius rather then as the show-off parlor trick it is. For, if we examine his function as a personal physician, we can see he needs a different orientation. He can no longer collect all his own raw data, although he must evaluate it. He must concentrate on his skill with nonverbal communication to assess a patient's symptoms. But he need not search out details of family history, past medical history, habits or employment unless they are pertinent to the present problem. His physical examination can be selective as long as it is completed by someone. His knowledge of disease processes becomes paramount; his skill in integrating the soft data of history and physical with the harder data of the laboratory becomes his central diagnostic chore.

In monitoring the operation of his treatment model, the physician needs hard data from laboratory and physical measurements plus his own sensitively acquired impressions of the patient's complaints and attitudes toward illness and recovery.

Thus, clinical associates or assistants can be used, as well as the technical and support professionals now available. The use of these paraprofessionals and physicians' assistants demands more managerial or executive skill than most physicians now develop. Also, it is quite clear from studies of their use that the physician's productivity may not go up in proportion to the volume of work done by the associate. When all a professional need do is think, he cannot work a 12-hour day. Thus, associates help increase productivity less than predicted.

Technical professionals, such as pathologists, radiologists and nuclear medicine specialists, represent a spectrum from near clinical orientation to frank laboratory workers. The overlap of clinical pathologists (MDs) with biochemists, bacteriologists, cytologists and others indicates the non-clinical nature of this group. They procure and interpret data for us, which still needs clinical interpretation.

Support professionals provide much-needed therapeutic assistance. Social workers, dietitians, physiotherapists and occupational therapists work with patients for generally narrow purposes. Administrators provide logistical support as well as reminding us of public concerns with our methods.

No one has conceptual difficulty with the place of technical or support professionals in the professional staff or health team of the future. The problem in the people-system lies with the clinically oriented health workers who will help the primary physician with individual, personalized and, yes, loving care of patients.

The nurse has been trained and, more recently, educated to assist in patient recovery from illness, in therapeutic procedures, in diagnostic data-gathering and in evaluating psychosocial factors in recovery. Case finding and health education have been added as specialized areas of nursing. Specialty treatment areas such as midwifery, anesthesia, surgical assistance, emergency room triage and rehabilitation nursing are now more common.

In the spectrum of skills described for the primary physician, the nurse most obviously lacks two important tools. The first is data-gathering by history and physical examination. And the second is sufficient knowledge of disease to build diagnosis and treatment models with confidence.

With nursing experience, history-taking experience and knowledge of common diseases are automatically expanded. The use and significance of laboratory data are partially acquired. Physical examination techniques are minimally learned. Nurses do acquire something else needed in the social art of primary medicine. By tradition and by precept, they usually develop a professional attitude of service, of the therapeutic use of one's self, of privileged communication, of dedication to the patient's welfare first. As cynical as the public may be about doctors and nurses, the bedside nurse still shows professional pride. This is important in primary care.

Therefore, I am involved in training "nurse clinicians," first as generalists, then if they wish, as nurse specialists. Our Regional Medical Program grant specifies recruitment from the urban ghetto and the rural areas so that we have a chance of sending help to physicians in those areas. Their training will be in history-taking, physical diagnosis, the significance of laboratory findings and in common disease processes. After didactic and practical sessions, they will be apprenticed to physician clinicians. Independent practice is some time away. They will have "eyeball," "over the shoulder" and direct supervision for a long time. They will always have telephone or radio and, hopefully, videophone supervision.

What of the Medex, the Physician's Assistant, the feldsher? I believe they can become primary physician associates, but it will take about the same length of time as a nurse. Now that we have more RNs, we can extend their training and produce physician associates faster than training *de novo*. The nurse is already accepted by physicians and by the public as a primary health resource. Only modest revision of nurse-practice acts or more liberal interpretation of supervision definitions need be sought.

More important, nurses themselves have finally realized that advancement lies more logically as clinicians, not administrators. Financial rewards must be generated; postgraduate clinical degrees must be awarded; and physician acceptance of the nurse as a colleague should be encouraged.

Much has been said and written about upward mobility in health careers. I agree in principle. I supervise a complete nursing career ladder at my hospital. However, I find it difficult to imagine the curriculum necessary to broaden and deepen the nurse clinician's or physician associate's knowledge sufficiently to satisfy requirements for medicine. For example, the core curriculum in nursing would have to be expanded greatly for nurses who expect to go on to medicine.

When physician assistants or nurse clinicians become primary care associates, there will still be all sorts of others in the advanced people-system.

Based on a core curriculum for practical nurses, many types of health care technicians can be trained. These individuals need mostly motor skills and can be assigned to functional areas of the health care system. We take high school graduates and, in four months of training, produce a general technician. We then train them as surgical technicians, emergency room technicians, orthopedic technicians, obstetrical technicians and as trainees in inhalation therapy, physical therapy and the lab. They have both lateral and upward mobility since they can enroll in local community college or medical technology school courses with some transferable credits.

The problem of credit transfer for our veterans plagues all of us. The quality of Armed Forces courses varies considerably. Recognition for certification, licensure or academic advancement is poor. Perhaps the Hebert bill in Congress, establishing a University of the Armed Forces, will help in the future.

The legal problems in the medical people-system have been compounded, I believe, by politicians. In my state a physician's assistant law has just been passed placing exact regulatory powers in the Health Department. An advisory committee with more politicians than physicians will define the assistants' practice limits. I believe any rules are premature.

Liberalization of nurse practice arts needs to allow more activity related to more education, training and experience. In New York, we had to stop our governor by hue and cry from signing a revised Nurse Practice Act which would have allowed any RN to diagnose and treat. The act was a good one, except for failure to provide for the nurse clinician as a new and more independent professional. Other states have passed laws forcing recognition of service schools for x-ray technicians, laboratory workers and LPNs.

I am not sure anyone knows what the elements of an advanced people-system should be. For the sake of our patients, I hope it is based on a sound educational job ladder, with adequate mobility and rewards to attract the best people we can get.

Health Evaluation in Transition

It is impossible to talk intelligently about "health evaluation in transition" without some understanding of the major forces that are buffeting and shaping the health care system as a whole and even the general economy.

The impact of the national wage-price freeze is just beginning to be felt in the health care industry. What will happen to the economy in general after the temporary freeze expires remains to be seen. The uncertainty is particularly great in our industry. Those who do not anticipate any permanent or fundamental change in U.S. economic policy point to the American people's historic opposition to economic controls in peacetime, a position which the President has repeatedly emphasized in the past, and which makes it difficult to be sure whether this represents a genuine change or just another in a long series of federal policy vacillations. Others claim that, even if a new policy of stabilization is developed for the general economy, the experience of World War II and Korea indicates that the health care industry will not be greatly affected.

Obviously, no one knows exactly what will happen after November 13. But the groundswell of Congressional and public support for the wage-price freeze, even from organized workers and from leading Democratic economists, suggests that our world will never be quite the same again. Moreover, 1971 is not 1941 or even 1951. The low prices, low wages and low profile of the health care industry which minimized the impact of government regulation during earlier control periods no longer prevail. On the contrary, the industry has now been singled out as one of the two most inflation-prone in the whole economy. It is also one of the largest, whether measured in terms of annual dollar volume or of employment, one of the most vital in terms of individual health and welfare, and was already marked for increased regulation even before the freeze.

It was considerations of this type which led me to advocate, over three years ago, that the industry proclaim a voluntary one-year freeze on all

---

Anne R. Somers, *Professor, Department of Community Medicine, College of Medicine and Dentistry of New Jersey, Rutgers Medical School, Piscataway, N. J.*

prices to be followed by a stabilization program of its own[1] — a move that might have obviated the need for national health insurance as well as saving the industry from its now highly exposed, highly vulnerable position.

That proposal is now ancient history. But once again, I urge the industry and its leaders not to gamble on the possibility of continuing "business as usual," but to face the probability that some form of economic stabilization will be continued after the temporary freeze expires and to take the lead in developing new policies appropriate to what Secretary of the Treasury Connally calls the new era when "American business and labor may have to get used to the idea of living within certain parameters."

The New Parameters

What are some of these new parameters that are likely to affect the health care industry? I believe there are at least four:

1. We are going to have to accept direct financial controls in one form or another. Whether this takes the form of a compulsory stabilization program for the economy as a whole, as in World War II, or more flexible and selective "guidelines," or special regulation of the health care industry — either as a substitute for or in addition to the general program — is still unclear. But that the industry — including most of its personnel — will be subject to some such regulation is now practically certain.

2. We can probably anticipate a much slower rate of growth than during the past decade. This is not only likely to result from less inflation — the major cause of the spectacular rise of the recent past — but from some cutbacks in utilization and perhaps even quality as well. This will not be an easy situation to live with. We have become accustomed to tremendous annual growth rates. But, as I see it, the new money simply isn't there. The tremendous federal budget deficits are forcing the Administration to think in terms of real austerity. The prospects for national health insurance now seem much dimmer for the immediate future. So do the prospects for continuing rises in private health insurance premiums.

3. Paradoxically, for at least part of the industry, the downward pressure on prices could be accompanied by upward pressure on wages. This will be particularly true if the World War II wage stabilization pattern — with tri-partite enforcement machinery — is followed after November 13. Historically, this approach resulted in substantial enhancement of union prestige and membership. The comparatively

low wage scales that still persist in some segments of the health industry will almost certainly present a tempting target for union leaders determined to correct "inequities" as well as to get something out of the new situation.

4. The combination of these three factors — price controls, tighter sources of new money, and increased union pressure on continuing low-wage occupations, all in the context of unremitting public attention — will inevitably result in much greater emphasis on productivity. This, as every health economist knows, is a concept that has never been adequately defined in the health services industry, let alone effectively cultivated. In plain language, however, higher productivity simply means doing more with fewer people. There will probably be increased public pressure to relate everything that is being done in the industry, and all the money that is being spent, to understandable indices of individual and national health.

Legislative and third-party judgments on these matters are likely to prove rather crude and even cruel at times. Employment in the industry will probably decline temporarily, rather than follow its long-run trend of growth. In some cases this will be the result of overdue tightening up on personnel policies and practices; in other cases, meat-ax budget cuts. The prospect for experimentation in the more esoteric aspects of medical practice and more expensive forms of rehabilitation also seem rather dim at the moment. The extent to which the negative aspects of this belt-tightening period can be mitigated and the opportunity for development of greater efficiency and new growth exploited will depend primarily on the quality of leadership demonstrated by the industry during the next year or two — especially during the next few months.

Some Basic Long-Term Issues

While we grapple with the immediate problems posed by the freeze and its sequelae, it would be a serious error to lose sight of the long-term problems and issues that have been building up for years and which will have to be faced — regardless of the economic temperature. These problems are by no means all economic; nor can they be solved by the industry alone apart from the rest of the economy. They constitute an agenda of ongoing business that will not be solved in the lifetime of any of us.

But broad and intractable as they are, the following nine issues seem to me to constitute the basic agenda to which all of us who aspire to positions of leadership must address ourselves now and for the foreseeable future — an agenda not superseded but on the contrary made more urgent by the new economic environment. Here is my list:

1. Consumer lifestyle and problems of health education.
2. Availability of 24-hour comprehensive care.
3. Rationalization of the delivery system.
4. Redefinition of professional roles to assure personalized care.
5. Free choice and consumer responsibility.
6. Quality controls.
7. Cost controls.
8. Long-range financing.
9. Long-term care, especially of the aged.

In view of time constraints it is obviously impossible to discuss all nine. I will confine myself to three which seem most relevant to the colloquium to which I have been assigned.

Consumer Lifestyle and Health Education

Few people would mention "lifestyle" as a major health problem but that is, in essence, what the poor are talking about when they beg for help with the drug problem, what the doctor means when he rails at the "irresponsibility" of his patients, or the third-party payer at "unreasonable" increases in utilization. Indeed, most of the nation's major health problems — including automobile accidents, all forms of drug addiction including alcoholism, venereal disease, obesity, many cancers, most heart disease, and most infant mortality — are primarily attributable not to shortcomings on the part of the providers but to living conditions, lifestyles, or ignorance of the consumer.

No amount of additional funding or even reorganization of the delivery system is likely to have much impact on this problem. On the contrary, additional funds for medical care, unless accompanied by effective educational measures, could actually contribute to further consumer irresponsibility, especially with respect to the promiscuous use of drugs, X-rays, and possibly some surgery.

The health-threatening aspects of affluence are just now beginning to be recognized. Even in Russia, where the standard of living is considerably lower, the syndrome which has been identified as "affluencia consumeritis" is reported to be spreading.[2,3] But we will have to do much more than simply identify this new health problem. Large-scale, nationwide programs of health education, family planning, health maintenance, and environmental management are needed. These may be difficult to implement. Not only may they conflict with present employment patterns, as the environmentalists are discovering to their distress, but with deep-rooted cultural patterns. The effort to cut down on smoking and on too much cholesterol intake often arouses the opposition not only of those who make their living in the tobacco and dairy products industries but of the potential victims themselves.

This complex issue will become even more so as we further socialize the costs of health care. The non-smoking taxpayer is likely to ask with increasing frequency why he should be taxed to finance medical care for a smoker while the latter dies a lingering expensive death from lung cancer or emphysema. But to impose a puritanical regime of non-health threatening foods and habits on an entire population would not only be politically impossible, as indicated by our experiment with prohibition, it would probably be scientifically impossible, and involve a threat to civil liberties. Some reconciliation between these points of view must be hammered out. The primary approach should be education, rather than regulation, although the latter will have to be used much more effectively than in the past.

Undoubtedly, what would help most of all would be a renewed sense of national purpose − a purpose that is meaningful to all segments of society − and of the individual's role in striving toward that purpose. Young people, in particular, but to a lesser extent all of us, are healthier as well as happier and more productive, when striving toward some goal which we feel is larger than ourselves. Without some such objective, we tend to lapse into health-threatening and often life-destructive habits and diversions of one kind or another. The personal self-discipline essential to a long and healthy life is inevitably related to the conviction that the game is worth the gamble.

Redefinition of Professional Roles to Assure Personalized Care

Both the need for, and the movement toward, some system of health care are indisputable. As already noted, systemization is not only inevitable but desirable. There is, however, a danger in this engineering approach − the danger that we become so enamoured with the challenge of systems-building or the efficiency of technological diagnosis that we forget one of the major purposes of it all − educating the patient to understand and to cope successfully with his health problems.

The challenge is to create a system that will give us the best of both worlds − the world of advanced science, technology, heavy capital investment, sophisticated management, specialized personnel, and systems engineering − but also the world of individual freedom, individual responsibility, respect for privacy and human dignity, understanding of the holistic or psychosomatic nature of health and disease, and appreciation of the need of human beings for other human beings.

It is not enough to pay sentimental tribute to the ideal family doctor, the "Marcus Welbys" of television make-believe and public yearning. We must now create the institutions and conditions to make it possible for real live doctors and other health professionals to be both scientists and humanists and to shift their primary attention from crisis intervention to lifetime prevention and health maintenance.

Three ways of dealing with this problem will be noted:

1. Revitalization of the doctor-patient relationship,
2. Development of new categories of health professionals,
3. Development of the concept of the health care team.

The patient's complaint as to the difficulty of establishing a meaningful doctor-patient relationship is probably the most widely expressed criticism of health care today. Some would-be reformers dismiss this complaint as sentimental nostalgia with no justification in this day of scientific medicine. It is true that the phrase "doctor-patient relationship" has been widely abused as a propaganda weapon in the futile effort to stave off third-party financing. If, as a result, the concept has lost its intrinsic meaning then it is high time that some real content be injected. For this widespread yearning has a firm basis in the realities of good medical care – in the instinctive realization that the patient must be viewed as a whole if effective management of his illness is to be achieved.

Just how this personal relationship can be maintained with a ratio of 770 potential patients for every practicing doctor and still permit these doctors to live a reasonably civilized life is obviously one of our major issues. The Kaiser plan claims to meet the need with one doctor for over a 1000 members and some people say the nation as a whole should be able to do almost as well.

I am a great admirer of the Kaiser system.[4] I consider prepaid group practice one of the most innovative concepts in health care this country has ever produced. But I do not consider it a panacea for all our problems. The low physician-population ratio depends in part on the atypical nature of the Kaiser membership. Moreover, as Kaiser officials have frequently pointed out, the physician shortage is one of the major obstacles to more rapid development of Kaiser-type organizations.

It is also true that enrollment in our medical schools has been increasing steadily for the past decade and the physician/population ratio is improving. Some fear that in another decade there will be too many doctors. Others say that the amount spent on medical education today is disproportionate to the national benefits accruing from such investment.

There is no question but that an oversupply of physicians is a possibility at some theoretical point in the future. I do not believe that point is yet in sight. But I do think that the large sums of public money now going for such education should be deliberately directed toward the expressed public demand for more primary doctors and for doctors who are willing and able to work with other health professionals in group settings so as to maximize their effectiveness.

The emergence of new health professions and occupations is already receiving a good deal of attention. "Physician's assistant," "Medex," "pediatric nurse practitioner," "child health associate," "rehabilitation coordinator" — these are just a few of the new job titles and job categories that are struggling to be born in one place or another. This is an exciting development. Once the omnipresent licensing and malpractice problems are cleared up and the training somewhat standardized, it could lead to a basic job category of "family health associate" and thus help to close the gap between supply and demand with respect to primary care.

Thus far, however, there is no agreement as to the major purpose of the new professions, except to relieve the immediate professional shortages. To avoid utter confusion and a serious threat to quality, much more thought needs to be given to the relationship of these new job categories and training programs to each other, to the older professions — not only the doctor but the nurse and pharmacist whose continuing indispensable roles are often overlooked — and to the very concept of the health care team. To develop the new categories, one by one, and seek to license them, one by one, would probably do more harm than good.

For some years, it has been fashionable to speak of the "team," thus paying at least lip service to the essential role of the dentist, the nurse, the pharmacist, the hospital administrator, the bioengineer, the medical economist, the social worker, the various therapists, aides, and others. In a few areas, teams do function effectively. Heart and brain surgeons often put together beautifully orchestrated teams of operating room personnel. In some hospitals "team nursing" has brought together the RN, the LPN, the aide, the ward clerk, and others. Perhaps the best example is in rehabilitation, where multidisciplinary teams, designed to get the patient from the operating table back to work, have produced miracles of recovery. OEO has pioneered, in some of its health centers, with primary care teams.

By and large, however, the concept of the health team remains largely a figure of speech. The health professions resemble more a hierarchy than a team. Most doctors and even nurses are individual entrepreneurs, in work habits even if not financially. The irony is that this extreme individualism instead of improving the patient-professional relationship, frequently makes a sound relationship impossible. The hurried, harried doctor or nurse, preoccupied with minutiae and mechanical details, cannot function as the wise, compassionate adviser. Who ever saw Marcus Welby in a hurry? What do we really mean by the health care team, especially in the area of primary care?

What is needed now is a variety of experiments along all the lines that have been suggested and others not yet thought of. These experiments should deal with the following:

1. An appropriate personal physician, with the competence, interest, and time to maintain a personal, continuing, and educational relationship with his patients — the sort of relationship that the fortunate minority now have with their pediatricians, internists, or obstetricians, but is unavailable to millions.

2. An effective physician-surrogate who could handle, for those unable to achieve such a relationship with a doctor, at least part of the personal aspects of health care.

3. Appropriate health care teams to deal with various types of patient populations and in various settings institutional and noninstitutional.

4. Appropriate use of computers, electronic monitoring and diagnostic aids, television, and other mechanical devices designed to increase the availability of health care, improve the quality, or reduce the cost.

While it is obviously easier to develop health care teams and their mechanical aids in an institutional setting, it is not necessarily the only way. Indeed, one of the big arguments for computerized medical records and intercommunity telediagnosis is, in my view, the fact that they make possible the desirable combination of centralized quality controls along with physical decentralization.

Regardless of setting, however, meaningful developments of this type will require simultaneous experimentation with new approaches to personnel licensing — an absolute prerequisite to solution of the health care crisis.

Free Choice and Consumer Responsibility

Consumer "free choice" is another important concept which has almost been reduced to a meaningless cliché as a result of propaganda overuse. Actually, the concept is basic to an effective health care system. People who are denied choice of health care programs or doctors are not likely to develop a responsible attitude toward the use or abuse of that care or even their own health. Free choice is an important factor in health maintenance.

Needless to say, it has to be reconciled with essential quality controls. People cannot claim the right to use quacks or to pursue illusory cancer cures at public expense. Even here, however, the boundaries are never clear-cut. In general, all persons, no matter how poor, should have the right to at least two *informed* options as to the type or system of health care they prefer. The uninformed "free choice" available to the middle class in some communities today is often less meaningful than the limited but informed choice between two or three types of health insurance available to most federal employees under the Federal Employees Health Benefits Program and to many industrial workers under collectively bargained contracts.

The technique of "dual choice" or "multiple choice" has worked reasonably well for employed persons and their families. It will be much more difficult to provide such choice to the poor whose standards are likely to be very unsophisticated. Nevertheless, this must be the goal. Any effort to assign poor people to programs that they consider unacceptable will inevitably be self-defeating. Since the Number 1 objective is to foster health education and a lifestyle conducive to good health there can be no compromise on this point.

The problem of "consumer control" is closely related. The drive for "consumerism," "Naderism," "participatory democracy," "decentralization," — whatever one wants to call it — is powerful, and in any case inevitable — given our commitment to universal education and universal suffrage. It is hard on the "Establishment" — particularly those conscientious segments that fear, probably correctly, that the quality of care may temporarily deteriorate under uninformed consumer pressures. But if we really believe that health is not something that can be given or bestowed by one individual to another, but has to be worked for and earned, then there is no turning back from this road. Consumers have to be brought into the decision-making process and brought in at the community or grass-roots level where it really matters in terms of their own health and where their experience can be — if intelligently used — an asset rather than a liability.

Administrative decentralization is obviously indispensable to achievement of this goal. The neighborhood health center movement — despite the frequency of political problems and the exorbitant costs — has been a healthy development. Not an end in itself — for the neighborhood center is even less capable of delivering comprehenisve care than the average community hospital — it has provided a training ground for thousands of disadvantaged persons in the complexities of health care policy-making and administration.

The effort on the part of some hospitals, for example, the Health and Hospitals Corporation of New York City, to establish community policy boards is equally significant.[5] When these various local efforts are eventually linked together into a viable regional health care system, with two-way communications between the local and regional centers, the educational value to all concerned may turn out to be even more important than the improvement in technical quality. The creators of the Regional Medical Programs had a vision of this utopia but academic elitism, combined with the general fear of change, has impeded its achievement. Perhaps the "comprehensive" health planners will move us further down this road.

The Future of Health Evaluation

By now, perhaps some of you are thinking that I have completely ignored my assigned topic — health evaluation in transition. True, I have not even mentioned the term "multiphasic screening." Partly this is because I know my limitations in the presence of experts such as Dr. Collen, Dr. Garfield, and many others. But chiefly this is because I have construed my assignment as one of helping to define the socioeconomic and political environment in which health evaluation will have to be developed along with other components of the evolving health care system.

I have tried to define some of the major factors in this rapidly changing environment — in terms of both immediate and long-term pressures. To recapitulate, the immediate pressures center about the nature of the economic stabilization program for the general economy, which will follow expiration of the temporary wage-price freeze, and any special regulation which may be applied to the health care industry. The long-term pressures center about the challenge of devising a health care system which combines the efficiency made possible by modern technology and specialization with the personal, individual, and humanistic values that are essential to the major purpose of the whole enterprise — educating the consumer to understand and cope with his own health problems.

Multiphasic screening, with its imaginative use of the most advanced technological equipment and multidisciplinary operational teams, with its potential for greatly reduced unit costs as well as impressive quality controls, has become not only a key element in the evolution of such a system, but a symbol of the entire system. In my view it constitutes a major breakthrough in the evolution of the health care system of the future.

But not everyone shares this view. There are many doctors as well as patients who see it as a massive "cop-out" — an effort on the part of overworked doctors to put a piece of machinery or a "paraprofessional" between them and "overdemanding" patients, an effort to dehumanize medicine. I am reminded of a prediction made by Dr. Oscar Creech, Jr., a distinguished surgeon at Tulane University School of Medicine, as to the future of medical practice *circa* 1990 which bears some resemblance to George Orwell's better known predictions regarding society in general *circa* 1984:

The private practice of medicine will no longer exist as we now know it. Physicians will be geographic full-time employees of the medical center complex, within which they will provide total medical care ... All diagnostic procedures and some parts of the physical examination, with the notable exceptions of the pelvic and rectal examinations we hope, will be performed automatically and interpreted by computer systems. The patient's entire medical record, from birth on, will be instantly available. Patients who require intensive care will be under constant observation of monitoring devices which, coupled with computers, will detect abnormalities and correct them automatically ... Medicine will be practiced on an assembly-line basis, but there is no reason to believe that patients will complain much about loss of the legendary doctor-patient relation. After all, no one has complained much about the disappearance of the personal attention we used to get from the grocer, baker, cleaner, and others who provide services in a community. It is therefore unlikely that the depersonalization of medicine will be noticed.[6]

Mechanized pelvic examinations and machines which not only detect abnormalities in intensely ill patients, but correct them as well, may or may not be an improvement over the fallible hand and head of the human doctor, in terms of some abstract definition of quality. My guess is that the very concept would be so unattractive to most patients and most doctors that they would end up by repudiating any system of advanced medical technology which attempted to use such devices.

Perhaps Dr. Creech's prophecies should not be taken too seriously. He is just one man. But already there *are* signs that the very concept of medical systems — the concept that underlies the existence of this organization — is in danger. Danger from those who would like to substitute the "system" for personal professional care and danger from those who fear that any "system" must result in such a substitution.

The current widespread criticism of screening — chiefly because the "yield" in terms of previously undetected disease may not seem worth the cost — seems to me to reflect such a misunderstanding. I find it tragic, as well as ironic, that Group Health Insurance of New York, a long-time proponent of preventive medicine in general and multiphasic screening in particular, has been forced to eliminate screening from its benefits for New York City employees at precisely the same time that a new state law is forcing it to cover chiropractic services. In fact, GHI is considering the elimination of screening examinations from its benefit package for all of its 1.3 million subscribers.

Before damning the state, the city, or the carrier for turning their backs on modern scientific medicine, the leaders of scientific medicine might ask themselves why the representatives of the public have taken these backward steps? Could it have something to do with the profession's seeming neglect of the entire field of primary care — a neglect that has forced many patients to turn to chiropractors, druggists, or even witch doctors? Could it be related to the effort in some quarters of the profession to turn the new patient over to the computer when what he wants more than anything else is to talk to another human being? What about the economics of screening? Are the savings, inherent in the high-volume, low unit-cost operation, passed on to the consumer either in terms of reduced health insurance premiums or better overall health care?

We stand at a fateful crossroads today not only in the field of health care but our whole technological society. Either we humanize the machine and harness its marvelous potential for strictly human purposes, or, like the old Luddites in the days when the Industrial Revolution first came to England, the people will destroy the machines and the systems for which they stand.

This organization — with its combined membership of physicians and engineers — may contain the clue to the future. science and technology in the service of humanity. Any attempt to reverse this formula, to reduce human beings — whether providers or consumers — to servants of science and technology — will inevitably fail.

References

1. Somers, A. R.: Doctors should declare a fee moratorium. *Medical Economics*, 45:23-40, 1968.
2. Russian sees threat in leisure, *N. Y. Times*, August 2, 1971.
3. Somers, A. R.: *Health Care In Transition: Directions for the Future.* Chicago: Hospital Research and Educational Trust, 1971, p. 21ff.
4. Somers, A. R.: Kaiser, HMO's, and the health care crisis, editor's preface, *The Kaiser-Permanente Medical Care Program: One Valid Solution to the Problem of Health Care in the U. S.* New York:Commonwealth Fund, 1971.
5. Action of the Health and Hospitals Corporation of New York in establishing the first hospital community board at Goldwater Memorial Hospital, *N. Y. Times*, August 5, 1971.
6. Creech, O., Jr.: Medical practice in 1990, *Bulletin of the Tulane University Medical Faculty*, 25:229-238, 1966.

The Critical Issue: Normal or Normative?

Dean F. Davies

A Presidential Address often looks backward with "pride" on the accomplishments of the organization, "views with alarm" the current scene and exhorts the audience about "closing ranks." Mine will discuss what I consider to be the critical issue.

My critical issue is not the public's concern about the economy or the health care crisis. It focuses on the theme of this Third Annual Scientific Meeting: "Health Evaluation: An Entry to the Health Care System." I want to re-examine with you the standards by which we evaluate the millions of pieces of information we, as physicians and as clinical engineers, as statisticians and as epidemiologists, are adding to the data base of hundreds of thousands of persons annually. The standards we use in evaluating the information that multiphasic health testing facilities dump onto cards, magnetic tapes, disc files and printouts are, of course, — you say — the normal values. And it is precisely the normal values that I propose to challenge.

I call it the critical issue because periodic health evaluation — automated or otherwise — is being challenged by pragmatists and rightly so.

The critical issue, in the sense of periodic health evaluation as any entry system to health care, is what we do with the data base after we get it. The interpretation hinges on how we select the reference point. When the statistician was asked "How is your wife?" and responded "Compared to whom?" he may have been more scientific than most of us would be under similar circumstances. He had to have a standard or a reference point. The fact is that — for certain reference points at least — we have all been wide of the mark. We have locked in on the mean plus or minus two or three standard deviations as the goal. We call the mean "normal" and think it is synonymous with "healthy." A few definitions are needed.

First, "normal" certainly does not mean free of disease. Eighty-five percent (85%) of the United States population over age 40 has periodontal disease. Most of us in this room have varying degrees of atherosclerosis. It does not mean ideal! It really represents the prevailing condition, the

Dean F. Davies, M.D., Ph.D., *Professor of Preventive and Community Medicine, University of Tennessee, Memphis, Tenn. Past-President, Society for Advanced Medical Systems.*

45

typical or common characteristics of a population. "Prevailing" because the data have to be defined in the context of both period of history and geographic and local conditions existing at the time.

I propose to relegate the use of normal values to their rightful position in the hierarchy of things. The issue is very clear. It is a question of no longer confusing what is the usual, customary, average, expected, prevailing or commonplace, on the one hand, with the ideal, the goal, the optimum, the heuristic, or the standard, in fact the norm, on the other. This mistake has been made century after century from Plato to modern times. Webster[1] reflects this confusion by including both concepts in his several definitions of "normal." In fact, while defining the word as "the usual state or condition" in one definition, within another normal is "not deviating from the common type of standard." During the Black Plague it was normal to die of the disease. If one of those normal atherosclerotic plaques I mentioned happens to be in a coronary artery and causes symptoms or a heart attack, then we are sick and that is abnormal. How capriciously we change the definition. One man can have advanced sclerosis of main arteries and be considered normal and another with a plaque in the wrong spot is abnormal. How anthropocentric can one get? Several of our customs need re-examination. It is the custom to define "normal" primarily on clinical grounds, based on the absence of symptoms. Secondarily it is a statistical definition based on frequency of occurrence.

The root word is "norm" (from norma, a carpenter's square),[1] clearly defined as a "model or example to be followed"; "a degree of quality that is proper and adequate for a given purpose"; "a standard." Norm has another adjective beside "normal"; it is normative; seldom used but it clearly refers to regulative or heuristic functions. "Normative science" is a science that "tests or evaluates." It is not merely descriptive. Just as the belief that the atom was the irreducible ground substance of matter has been replaced by demonstrations of numerous subatomic products; so the concept that "normal" is to be equated with the "ideal" or healthy state has to give way to scientific evidence. We can do better than to use the prevailing condition as a standard of health.

In a delightful but scholarly spoof on the word "normal," the astute physiologist, Homer Smith,[2] attributed the confusion of the "normal" with the "ideal" to Plato. After decimating Plato for this, he proceeded to show that the more we seek to describe a "normal" person statistically as the ideal or paradigm, the further we get removed from anything meaningful He wound up calling the Clementine of "Oh, My Darling Clementine" his paradigm while showing that her "herring boxes without topses" and other characteristics were anything but normal.

Our Customs

What are our customs which have served us satisfactorily in the past but need to be replaced in the light of new insights into disease processes and new opportunities to use more sophisticated statistical methods?

The first custom in need of re-examination is the human desire to simplify. If it is too complex for the human mind to grasp, we cut it down to size. It is either good or bad; right or wrong; healthy or sick; normal or abnormal. On television shows we see life simplified to "the good guys" and "the bad guys." This we call *dichotomization*. But the closer we look at the healthy or the normal, the more they disappear. "The normal is gone because it never was."[2]

The second custom we have fallen into is being satisfied that clusters of homogeneity (normal distribution curves) are normal and that any heterogeneity will show up in a bimodal curve.[3] In doing so we fail to realize that there is no true homogeneity but only an infinite series of heterogeneities within homogeneities. The curve that represents people is made up of curves for males and females. Each can be divided into distribution curves for white and non-white, and examined for differences by age, height, weight and so on *ad infinitum*.

It is the custom of many of our laboratories, particularly commercial laboratories, to give a single range of values for "normal people" regardless of age, sex or race. This custom we call *homogenization*. Everyone knows that prevailing cholesterol values vary both by sex and age. But that complicates our lives enormously.

Our third custom is that of *anthropocentrism*. There is nothing in the natural world that distinguishes the normal from the diseased. In his play *The Family Reunion*, T. S. Eliot has Dr. Warburton saying, "We're all of us ill in one way or another: We call it health when we find no symptom of illness. Health is a relative term."

David Seegal[4] said almost ten years ago: "The physician would be quick to admit that sometimes he has less certainty in certifying the normal than the abnormal state of an organ or system."

Two years ago Cotlove[5] from George Williams' laboratory said, ". . . the problem of defining the normal versus the abnormal can become a serious public health problem in terms of economics and medical manpower." This is the issue with which we are faced. To justify periodic multiphasic health testing we must show, in quantifiable terms, how much death and disability can be prevented among presumably well persons without unwarranted cost of follow-up of false-positive suspects, on the one hand, or creating unjustified confidence among false-negative persons (with a disease), on the other. The ultimate question is one of cost-benefit.

The thoughtful statistician, Donald Mainland,[6] expressed the same thought in a discourse on normal values in medicine. He said that deciding what subjects should be selected for inclusion in the standard series is a much more difficult thing than deciding where to make cut-off points. Getting sick is as much a part of the natural or normal world as being well. Death is a normal phenomenon. Our goals have been shifting from concern about sickness — *feeling* sick[7] — to concern about risk factors for premature morbidity or death. To say that a physician's role should be limited to the sick is to perpetuate crisis medicine (and incidentally to keep the costs of health care soaring). At best it is medical hedonism and at worst it is medical myopia. There will be those who challenge me on that statement. I will stand with Max Planck[8] who said: "A new scientific truth does not triumph by convincing its opponents and making them see the light, but rather because its opponents eventually die, and a new generation grows up that is familiar with it."

Another of our habits which requires re-examination and is practiced widely, I call *Gaussianism*. The mean plus or minus two standard deviations become the standard, true or ideal value. Mainland describes Gaussianism as an addiction.[6,9] Since it becomes statistically difficult to handle skewed (un-symmetrical) distributions, we may set up an arbitrary rule to eliminate statistically what are called "outliers" after first selecting our "normal" population on a clinical basis. Efforts to identify the "normal" population vary from testing a few laboratory workers who happen to be around to carrying out a fairly thorough history and physical examination on a randomized population. The classical case of "normal" values being published on the basis of a minimum amount of data is reflected in the following statement made by Wintrobe[10]: "The values which have so long been cited for the normal red cell count in men and women, 5,000,000 and 4,500,000 per cu mm respectively, are based on determinations made more than a century ago on four subjects."

In any case, statistical manipulation is simply an admission that we have not been able by biological means to identify the normal. The reasoning, to me, is *rationalization* (I could say sophistry). If a statistical approach can identify heterogeneity, then it is not necessary to use clinical means. Otherwise, there is no biological basis to say that a value beyond two or three standard deviations is abnormal or from a different population or less desirable than others. Indeed, it may be super-normal. We forget that a skewed distribution is certain evidence of heterogeneity regardless of the presence of outlying values or bimodal distributions.

One other custom deserves mention, although some have been well aware of its pitfalls. To them I apologize for stressing the obvious. I call it *perseveration* in always thinking and reporting in terms of so many standard deviations encompassing the "normal" as if that cut-off had some intrinsic value. In terms of decision levels the cut-off point should be at that balance of false-positive and false-negative results (or sensitivity and specificity) that is best for that particular circumstance. Are you going to operate on the liver? You had better not have too many false positives — operating and finding a normal liver. If you merely want to narrow down to a manageable number of persons on whom to obtain a more precise secondary test, you can set a high sensitivity level (with several false suspects on primary screening). You can eliminate most of them by carrying out an acceptable secondary test.

Facts and Values

Now I would like to return to the question of normal versus normative. Normal is descriptive of what exists. Normative is a standard or goal. It makes a value judgment. The late Abraham Maslow said in his Karen Horny Memorial Lecture[11] that "Facts create oughts! The more clearly something is seen or known, the more ought-quality it acquires."

I dare say that most of us were brought up on the separateness of scientific truth or natural law and religious truth which encompasses morals and ethics. Maslow is suggesting that the value structure can be built on scientific facts. He is not alone.

Warren Weaver[12] described the unity of the universe in a different way. He said: ". . . the ultimate unifying virtues are order, beauty, faith, and love. The emphasis in science is upon the first of these four words, slowly tapering off on the remaining three. The emphasis of religion increases from first to last, culminating on the final word."

Kaplan[13] also recognizes the pursuit of values as grist for the scientist's mill. He recognizes intrinsic values (such as nourishment, shelter and education). Certainly as long as we remain relatively free of conflicts between interacting and conflicting value systems, we will be on safe ground.

Weight and Mortality

You will recall that I defined "normative science" as one that "tests or evaluates." One of the pioneers in this field was Louis Dublin, Medical Director of the Metropolitan Life Insurance Company for many years. Among the discoveries he made was the fact that those policy holders of average (or normal) body weight had a higher mortality rate than those who would be considered underweight by prevailing standards.[14,15] The normal was, therefore, not the norm or normative when measured in the context of life expectancy.

Heretofore, for the most part, we have taken the normal, average, prevailing condition as synonymous with the optimum state of health. I call it the *Apotheosis of the Mean* – the extreme exaltation of the prevailing, normal, or average condition.

It was in the enlightened self-interest of the Metropolitan Life Insurance Company – and incidentally for the public in general – for Dublin to establish new tables of ideal or "desirable" weights for each height.[15] They have blanketed the country.

They disregard age on the basis that adults should not put on weight on growing older, but they do allow us to decide whether we have a small, a medium, or a large frame. I have not discovered any quantitative definitions of small, medium and large frame. However, even the highest allowable weight for a large frame is usually below the average weight found in our population.

The Society of Actuaries pooled data from several insurance companies and published results in *Build and Blood Pressure Study* in two volumes. The mortality rates of these policy-holders rose for each age, sex and height-specific category directly as the weight increased. The presumably under-weight persons lived longer. It became interesting to speculate how much overweight the U.S. population is in terms of mortality. According to the Desirable Weight Tables,[15] a man 5′8″ with a medium frame should weigh 145 pounds. A 40-year-old man with these same height and weight characteristics in the general population has a mortality rate of 3.04/1,000, according to data derived from the study. The average weight of male policy-holders 40 years old and 5′8″ is not 145, but 163.[16] He is already 18 pounds over-weight in terms of life expectancy.

But policy-holders are not the average U.S. citizen. Fortunately, the National Health Survey has studied a number of characteristics of a carefully selected sample of the U.S. population including weight. The average 40-year-old American male of 5′8″ weighs 170 pounds.[17]

By making the assumption that differences between the U.S. male population and policy-holders are not weight-dependent, one can estimate the degree of association between excess weight *per se* and excess mortality in the country at large. It seems that the mortality rate of the average (5′8″, 170 pound) 40-year-old American male is not 3.04, but 3.65/1,000, or 20% above that expected of the same man weighing only 145 pounds. The data are, at best, first approximations.

To attach cause-effect significance to this association between weight and mortality requires a different kind of evidence. Though not epidemiologically clean, there is some evidence that reduction of weight will be accompanied by a reduction in mortality. With reduced premiums as an incentive, a large number of life insurance policy-holders reduced their weights and were given standard policies. These persons were followed for mortality rate over a period of years and it was discovered that the mortality among those policy-holders was markedly lower than among those who did not reduce.[16] This was also noted in an earlier study by Dublin and Marks.[18]

Of course, the possible effects of self-selection have to be ruled out, but it does not seem reasonable that the healthier men would decide to reduce any more than those with a disease to worry about.

Blood Pressure and Mortality

Upper limits of so-called normal ranges of blood pressure have been arbitrarily set at 140 mm Hg systolic and 90 diastolic. However, it is most interesting to note that data derived from the *Build and Blood Pressure Study* showed that the mortality rate of 40-year-old men near the upper level of this normal range (135/87.5) is 55% higher than those whose blood pressure is less than 115/70 mm Hg.[16] The definition of normal blood pressure is not a clinical one since much higher pressures exist without signs or symptoms. The normal or prevailing range again, as with body weight, is not normative; it should not be assumed to be optimal or ideal. The Veterans Administration Study[19] has clearly shown that the control of borderline and mild hypertension reduces the number of morbid events.

Cholesterol and Mortality

One other example, even though it is familiar, deserves to be mentioned. It is the serum cholesterol level. Some of the commercially available charts have taken normal (average, prevailing) values from the literature and show a range from 150 to 300 mg percent as being normal. On examining the relationship of cholesterol to mortality in the Framingham Study,[20] it was demonstrated that the mortality of 40-year-old men with a cholesterol of 300 mg percent is 2½ times that of men of the same age with a cholesterol of 210. The normative value for a population, in terms of life expectancy, is around 210 mg percent or perhaps lower.

Normative in Context of an Objective

So much for body weight, blood pressure, and cholesterol. Do normal values always differ from normative values? What about the electrolytes? In this case the homeostatic mechanisms are so delicate — indeed exquisite — that the analytic methods make up a considerable part of the coefficient of variation for repeated tests on the same individual; that is, of the coefficient of intra-individual variation. In short, our methodologies have not been perfected sufficiently to provide the precision required to distinguish between minor changes in values; certainly this is true of sodium and chloride ions.

The normative value in this case should be defined, until better evidence presents itself, as the average serum level of *each* individual around which the value fluctuates. It would be defined according to the individual's prevailing state rather than in terms of group averages. For the present no correlation with mortality rates has been recognized.

Please note that in each case the normative value is expressed in terms of some specific criterion other than that of conformity to the group average. Normative life styles will thus differ from prevailing life styles if measured in terms of a state-of-health index or of life expectancy. Health hazards of smoking, of high-saturated-fat diets, of alcoholism, and of lack of exercise are becoming quantifiable. The normative science is well on its way. The major stumbling block in its way is that of confusing what is normal, prevailing or average with what is optimum, ideal, heuristic or normative.

But there is one other stumbling block and it is a serious one. As much as we may fight for life after landing in the hospital with a serious illness, in the absence of symptoms, we act as if we believe that the length of our lives is not important. We constantly take unnecessary risks both actively and passively. There seem to be things more important than health or life itself. Either that or those who have the facts have not made us fully aware of the risks.

The question which faces medicine, particularly the primary physician, is how to help the individual know his risks and to achieve his goal — whatever he considers normative for him. It may not be length of life, but it is liable to be health. With the help of the engineer, the epidemiologist and the statistician, the physician can establish normative values for each individual. This is the ultimate in the doctor-patient relationship because the physician ministers to what both Paul Tillich[21] and Nels Ferré[22] call the "Ultimate Concern."

What is our Ultimate Concern? Are we humanists, hedonists, humanitarians or theists? Hopefully, the health professional will not dictate our values to us but he can help, as he ministers to our health, to work out a program — a life style — which seeks our personal, normative goals.

Conclusion

In fulfillment of the expected, I look backward with pride on the successes of the Society for Advanced Medical Systems but view with alarm the dichotomization and homogenization of data; the anthropocentrism, Gaussianism, rationalization, and perseveration in handling data; and above all, I view with alarm the apotheosis of the mean, exalting the normal to an undeserved pedestal.

Lastly, I implore both members and friends of this Society to close ranks in the construction of tables of normative values for every test and for every characteristic of life style which threatens life. I am happy to report that a small beginning has been made to this end.

This is what SAMS is all about: to enhance human values.

Acknowledgment

James Tchobanoff, A.M.L.S., assisted in library searches and statistical derivations. Harry Robinson, D.Sc., reviewed the statistical assumptions entailed in estimates of mortality rates.

References

1. *Webster's Third New International Dictionary of the English Language; Unabridged.* Springfield, Mass.:Merriam, 1961, p. 1540.
2. Smith, H. W.: *Bull. N.Y. Acad. Med.*, 23:352, 377, 1947.
3. Murphy, E. A.: *J. Chronic Dis.*, 17:301, 1964.
4. Seegal, D.: *JAMA*, 182:1031, 1962.
5. Cotlove, E., in Benson, E. S. and Strandjord, P. E. (eds.): *Multiple Laboratory Screening*, New York:Academic Press, 1969, p. 217.
6. Mainland, D.: *Ann. N.Y. Acad. Sci.*, 161:527, 1969.
7. Garfield, S. R.: *Sci. Amer.*, 222:15, 1970.
8. Planck, M.: *Scientific Autobiography, and Other Papers*, F. Gaynor (trans.). New York:Philosophical Library, 1949.
9. Mainland, D.: *Clin. Chem.*, 17:267, 1971.
10. Wintrobe, M.: *Clinical Hematology*, ed. 5. Philadelphia:Lea and Febiger, 1961, p. 104.
11. Maslow, A. H.: Fusions of facts and values. *Amer. J. Psychoanal.*, 23:117, 1963.
12. Weaver, W.: *Saturday Review*, 49:12 (May 28), 1966.
13. Kaplan, A.: *The Conduct of Inquiry: Methodology for Behavioral Science* (San Francisco:Chandler, 1963), quoted by Churchman, C. W.: *Science*, 147:283, 1965.
14. Dublin, L. I., Lotka, A. J. and Spiegelman, M.: *Length of Life: A Study of the Life Table*, rev. ed. New York:Ronald Press, 1949, pp. 193-196.
15. Dublin, L. I.: *Factbook on Man: From Birth to Death*, ed. 2. New York:Macmillan, 1965, pp. 301, 359.
16. *Build and Blood Pressure Study, 1959*, Chicago:The Society of Actuaries, 1959, vol. 1, pp. 17, 117-120.
17. Weight by height and age of adults, United States, 1960-1962, in *Vital and Health Statistics*, series 11, number 14. U.S. National Center for Health Statistics, 1966, p. 11.
18. Dublin, L. I. and Marks, H. H.: *Trans. Assn. Life Insurance Dir. Amer.*, 35:235, 1951.

19. Veterans Administration Cooperative Study Group on Antihypertensive Agents, *JAMA*, 213:1143, 1970.

20. *The Framingham Study: Epidemiological Investigation of Cardiovascular Disease*, (Superintendent of Documents, Washington, D. C., 1968-1970) sections 1-22.

21. Tait, L. G.: *The Promise of Tillich.* Philadelphia:Lippincott, 1971, pp. 32-34.

22. Ferré, N. F. S.: *The Universal World: A Theology for Universal Faith.* Philadelphia:Westminister Press, 1969, pp. 87-88.

Technology's Role in Health Evaluation

John R. Kernodle

To find the role technology will play in health care in the years ahead, we only have to look at the overall health objectives for the 1970s. These objectives can be summarized as follows: (1) making it easier for the patient to have access to medical and health care, (2) finding ways to emphasize early detection and treatment of disease, (3) improving the quality as well as increasing the quantity of care available, (4) finding the causes and the cures for disease, and (5) reducing the costs of care.

All of these objectives call for more and better efforts to develop new and better approaches to health care.

It stands to reason that in finding a beginning for these efforts, the logical first step in providing total health care is to improve the techniques and results of initial evaluation and diagnosis.

Evaluation and diagnosis are the road map and steering wheel for the journey into health care. If that trip is not begun in the right direction, the desired destiny is not likely to be reached. There is little doubt in my mind that technology — in the form of advanced systems of health evaluation — will play a dynamic role in the new era of total health care.

The process of health evaluation is a common and fundamental task within medicine. While it presents a great challenge, it also offers great promise to those of us who are looking for better ways to provide better patient care. It is the starting point in the traditional physician-patient relationship, and its continuing accuracy is necessary for continued patient management. There is no more appropriate area for the development of advanced methodology to help physicians in taking care of their patients. Significant steps have already been taken to apply technology to health evaluation. Any number of examples could be cited, such as the familiar automated multiphasic health testing, with its complex array of medical instrumentation and computer hardware designed to measure and record a variety of patient data.

Other systems in use or in various stages of development include monitoring and life support systems in hospital operating rooms and

John R. Kernodle, M.D., *Chairman, Board of Trustees, American Medical Association, and Chairman, AMA Committee on Computer Systems in Medicine, Chicago, Ill.*

55

coronary and intensive care units, computer diagnostic systems to help physicians identify a broad range of disorders and diseases, and automated laboratory systems that can perform dozens of tests very quickly. The examples mentioned are all part of the health evaluation process and, of course, there are many more systems of that type.

Most of us are well aware of the clinical benefits that can be gained through the use of those systems in medicine. No one will say there are no problems associated with their use. But whatever the problems might be, they are more than offset by the potential rewards if they are used correctly.

A question that might reasonably be asked is "What exactly are the benefits to be gained through the use of technology in health evaluation?" There are four good answers:

1. The effective use of technology can save time and manpower.
2. It can make available skills even more skillful.
3. It can improve efficiency.
4. It can help distribute services more effectively.

Through computers, a variety of functions can be monitored and controlled, thus freeing physicians and allied health personnel to do other things that require their attention. This is true whether we are talking about multiphasic testing, physiological monitoring, laboratory analysis or almost any other form of health evaluation.

At the office level, automated systems such as the multiphasic health testing devices can help physicians to see more patients or to better manage an already heavy patient load. This was demonstrated some time ago by a Public Health Service project that evaluated the use of automated medical histories and it was done in a five-man group practice. By collecting the history through automation, physicians saved from 20 to 30 minutes of every hour allotted to new patient work-up. Saving time through a technological approach can be really significant – since time is something that most of us involved in health care have very little of because of growing demands for our services.

By automating or systematizing certain functions, allied health people can also be used to greater advantage in performing jobs that do not require the presence of a physician. We can improve organization, heighten efficiency and increase productivity in many areas, including appointment scheduling, collection of patient history and chief complaints, physical testing, laboratory analysis, medical record-keeping and patient follow-up. Physicians can be in a better position to treat patients because they have more data for review and consideration – details that are collected before he ever sees or examines his patient. All of that can be made possible through effective distribution of jobs and sound management of data, which can be incorporated in the system.

Consider, too, the potential for technology in plans that are now emerging for organizing the personnel and facilities for health care. Such plans come in many forms, from both the public and the private sectors. Some are good, and some are bad, but most of them have at least one thing in common: emphasis on more preventive and ambulatory care. If such care can be significantly increased, it will undoubtedly demand more use of computerized health evaluation systems.

Traditional medical records, for example, will take on new meaning and have new value. In the past, fragmentary notes representing a patient's total medical history have been scattered through every doctor's office and hospital the patient has ever been in. In the future, it is possible that all of the fragments will be put together into one automated medical record. Just think of the clinical value it would have if a patient's complete history — all of the scientifically documented information from all the sources of care during his life — could be available to an attending physician for his review. Actually, it is not as far-fetched as it might sound. There are already several projects of that type — both in this country and abroad. In the projects, automated medical records are being developed for both community and regional medical information systems. Some are also collecting demographic information, such as birth, marital and death statistics, as well as other data about the community or region. The result will be comprehensive records, describing not only clinical characteristics of individuals but also sociological and environmental factors that can affect the health of individuals and of the community as a whole. A great deal of work remains to make such systems fully workable, but some day I believe they will be common. They will be the basis on which other medical systems are built.

Indeed, the make-up and design of those systems will be coordinated with overall national health objectives and will most likely become the framework in which efforts to reach total health objectives are carried out. That can only be done through technology. It can only be done through the combined efforts of dedicated people, computers, medical instrumentation and other factors brought together and guided by effective systems planning.

With continued planning, development and application of health evaluation systems, we will be in a better position to bring about improved overall health in this country. Through careful health evaluation and preventive care, we can lower morbidity and mortality. Through analysis of data on whole population groups, we can stimulate sociological and biomedical research. By coordinating all of the systems, we can clearly identify priority areas for better health planning.

In the long run, improvements in the level of health will lead to a reduction in the cost of health care. It's just as simple as this: If you keep more patients out of the hospital, you generate a tremendous national saving. And at the office level, savings can result from fewer patient visits for treatment of chronic disease and less need for long-term medication and therapy.

Before all of that can be done, however, there are some very real and very important issues which have to be settled. In developing automated systems, the first and most important criterion must be reliability. We are not talking about just correlating data or handling figures. We are talking about systems that deal with human lives. There can be no margin for error where the read-out of a computer will make a difference in the kind of care a patient receives, or worse, a difference in whether he receives any care at all and whether he lives or dies.

We cannot accept in this field the funny stories about computer errors such as the one that sent 47,000 copies of *Time* to one subscriber. There is nothing amusing about the idea of a computer reporting a wrong result of a laboratory test. It is not enough to develop automated or computerized systems just to make them available. It must be clear that they have positive advantages over other approaches to health evaluation and their use must have the support of physicians in the community. To get such support, the developers of systems will have to work closely with physicians who will use them, as well as with local and state medical societies, specialty organizations and others, to assure that the systems meet the needs of the physicians and do the jobs for which they are designed.

Another issue to be considered is the cost, regardless of the type of system − whether for physiological monitoring, automated multiphasic health testing or any other − the operating costs can be extremely high. To be self-sustaining, they must be designed to handle patient loads of sufficient size to keep the unit cost low; otherwise the possible savings mentioned earlier will all be lost.

Still another consideration is that the systems must, by design, be consistent, up to date and exhaustive. They also must be expedient, efficient and scientifically sound. Their effectiveness will be judged on their ability to trigger other activities within the overall health care system. In other words, they must play their role in improving quantity, quality and continuity of health care throughout the community. The problems will be solved, however. The growing demand for services and the consequent demand for more efficiency and productivity in health care leave little doubt that technology will be applied to health evaluation at a rapid rate. Indeed, rather than an absence of health evaluation techniques, the problem could very well become one of run-away development. It is important, therefore, that steps be taken now to make sure that technology in health evaluation will be used to its very best effect.

One necessity is for education. Medical students can be taught to use technology as a common tool in health evaluation. Practicing physicians can be made aware of potential improvements through continuing medical education. Special courses can be conducted for allied personnel.

Finally, as important as any of the other, patients can be encouraged to accept new evaluation procedures and techniques through various forms of public education. Standards for evaluating the reliability and effectiveness of existing and future technological methods must be continually reviewed and improved. Ethical as well as clinical guidelines must be maintained to assure dignity for the patient and integrity for the personnel involved in the health evaluation process. Privacy of patient information must be assured.

In addition, ways must be set up to identify and eliminate ineffective or undesirable developments in the application of technology. Those methods of identification and elimination must contain actual means by which such undesirable activity can be ended. Model projects can provide new insight into the potential role of technology. Any number of approaches can and should be tested and evaluated to check logistical as well as clinical aspects of health evaluation systems. Another important area for our attention is health care legislation.

We should make sure that legislative leaders understand the possible importance of technology in health care, with special emphasis on both the logistical and clinical advantages that are available to the physician, to the patient and to the third-party fiscal agent, where appropriate.

There are many other areas that call for attention. The need for continued, careful planning is obvious. However, we are fortunate in having in this country the intellectual resources, the interest and the capability to meet the challenges associated with the use of technology.

I am convinced that tremendous strides can be taken to meet the health care needs of all Americans. Effective coordination of our collective energy, however, is of paramount importance and that, as I see it, is the underlying goal of the Society for Advanced Medical Systems. Through this organization, the efforts of physicians, scientists, engineers and others can be channeled into the most productive directions. Fragmentary, isolated development of parts that might not fit into the whole picture can be minimized through the cooperation of all involved professional groups. The American Medical Association is eager to participate in this important work and to contribute to the continuing development of useful and valuable technology. We are confident that such contributions — by us and by others — can be truly meaningful to the future of health care.

In closing, I would like to offer one more thought on the subject of technology and health evaluation. It is simply this. If I had to choose one area of concentration for planning and developing technological systems in medicine, the choice would be an easy one. It would be in the process of health evaluation, in its many forms. For regardless of the degree to which we develop our talents in other areas of medicine or how prepared we are to undertake appropriate therapy, we must first be able to recognize the signs of illness, consider the possible variables and define the exact medical problem. The medical profession endorses any efforts that will help us do that job.

AMHT in the Metropolitan Hospital

Harry Hochstadt

Cedars of Lebanon Health Care Center is a changing hospital in a changing environment. Advances in technology have forced change on society, requiring a corresponding change in health care delivery. As a voluntary, non-profit hospital, located in metropolitan Miami, Florida, currently undergoing a $72 million expansion program, Cedars clearly sees its role in meeting the requirements of the changing health care delivery system.

One of the features of the new facility will be an automated multiphasic health testing laboratory. Our decision to include the automated health testing laboratory was reached in November 1969 after many months of research by our management staff. Our rationale was to use the automated health testing laboratory as a vehicle for mass patient flow into the health care system and to more effectively render service to patients being admitted to our hospital. The Board of Directors of the hospital authorized the automated health testing laboratory, providing the Medical Staff of the hospital would recommend it, and the Medical Staff gave a unanimous resolution to support the project.

Our research had indicated, at least to us, that to be most successful, a screen such as we envisioned had to be tailored to our local patient and physician population. Accordingly, the Medical Staff appointed a multi-disciplined Medical Advisory Committee comprised of 17 physicians to work with Medical Scientific International Corporation, the company selected to manufacture the automated health testing laboratory. The Committee and Medical Scientific International Corporation decided upon the specific tests to be performed and also developed the medical history questionnaire and printout.

The system selected by Cedars had a number of unique features in addition to having test batteries for both in- and out-patient. It is the hospital's intent to process most ambulatory in-patient admissions through the automated health testing laboratory, as well as providing test batteries for large employee groups, insurance company physicals, executive

Harry Hochstadt, *Executive Vice-President, Cedars of Lebanon Hospital, Miami, Fla.*

physicals and physician referrals. The manufacturer of the system states that when the system is installed, it will be the largest and fastest pre-test automated health testing laboratory ever constructed. The fourteen test stations and support locations contain 28 real-time terminals, 22 of which are cathode ray display terminals of four different designs. Test data are transmitted to and from the dual processor data control center at 9600 baud; therefore, the average response time from pick-up to the displayed result is only half a second!!

The total system is itself comprised of four subsystems, and it is compatible with some of our long-range plans for a real-time medical information network. The modules in the automated health testing laboratory are the automated processing system, the automated medical history and psychological system, the automated clinical laboratory and the automated screening system.

It is interesting to note that the automated clinical laboratory system not only provides load listing and in-process sample detection, but it also performs its own calibration of the clinical instruments. The automated medical history system is available in either Spanish or English by the patient and contains a psychological audit of the patient which is a subset of the M.M.P.I., developed by professionals in the field.

Subsystems

The clinical screening system is equipped with seven cathode ray tube (CRT) terminals for the entry and/or verification of test data, four automated log-on devices for monitoring patient test status in module, and the necessary automated medical instrumentation for performing measurements on the following parameters: height, weight, skinfold thickness, blood pressure, pulse rate, temperature, audio acuity, pulmonary function, visual acuity, tonometry, electrocardiogram, chest x-ray and thermography. The first eight tests are automated and on-line to the computer, i.e., test data transmitted directly from the test instrument to the computer without any operator intervention. The 12-lead electrocardiogram, chest x-ray and thermograph are interpretation tests — the interpretation comments being entered into the computer via mark-sense forms and document reader. The remaining tests, performed with automated instrumentation, require the technician to manually enter the test data via a CRT terminal.

The *clinical laboratory* is equipped with four CRT terminals for data entry and/or verification; four automated log-on devices for monitoring patient specimen status; and a printer for generating loadlist, interim reports on test result data and laboratory test status reports. The module also contains the necessary laboratory instrumentation for performing the following tests: a 12-parameter blood chemistry profile, a four-parameter electrolyte profile, a seven-parameter hematology profile, a three-parameter coagulation profile, protein bound iodine, tri-glycerides, reagin test, latex fixation, stool guaiac, pap smear, maturation indices, and urinalysis. The first seven of the above tests are automated with the 12-parameter blood chemistry profile being on-line to the computer. The remaining tests are manually performed, and the result data are entered into the computer via a CRT terminal.

The *medical history* section is composed of 11 CRT terminals specially designed to facilitate patient ease in responding to multiple choice and true-false questions. The patient responds to computer-generated medical history and psychological questions. If a patient's response to a particular medical history question is positive, the computer will generate additional, more specific questions pertaining to that particular subject area.

The *central processing* hardware configuration consists of a dual processor organization. Each processor has a dedicated system function to perform. The function of the primary (host) processor is to provide overall system management and control as well as to perform all patient data processing. The function of the secondary (communication) processor is to provide a telecommunication-compatible system interface for 31-character-oriented data terminals as well as to manage all message traffic between the host processor and the data terminals.

The capacity of the system is guaranteed to accomodate a minimum of 100 examinees in a normal eight-hour day and the system will provide 47 test parameters. The design is such that the test battery is entirely flexible to meet the requirements of the Medical Staff for changing needs. All results produced by the automated health testing laboratory will be sent to a referring physician, or in the case of in-patients being admitted, to the patient chart.

The automated health testing laboratory will be housed in the ground floor of our new South Building, which will also contain a comprehensive diagnostic clinic designed to accomodate 200 patients per eight-hour day. This has been planned so that the hospital can, if it so elects, establish a health maintenance organization and more effectively fulfill its role as a comprehensive health care center.

At the present time, it is anticipated that the charge for the complete battery of tests will be in the range of $85.00 to $100.00 per examinee. Each examinee should be able to complete the entire test battery in approximately 2 hours 20 minutes, and in the case of in-patients being admitted to the hospital, the test results will accompany the patient to the room and be inserted in the patient's chart. It is our expectation that a minimum of a half day's patient stay can be saved by all ambulatory in-patients being processed through the automated health testing laboratory. This in itself should reduce hospital costs. As of this date, the automated health testing laboratory is approximately 80% completed. In the interim, our hospital is finalizing its plans for marketing and education of our physician community. Much work still has to be done and we are not that naive whereby we expect the automated health testing laboratory to be an instant success in all aspects.

As a metropolitan health care center, Cedars views the hospital based automated health testing laboratory as a key and integral element in the organization of a new comprehensive medical delivery system to insure the changing needs of our community and professions.

The Potential Role of AMHT in Evaluation of HMOs

Harry E. Emlet, Jr.

The purpose of the paper is to focus attention on a new role which AMHT might well serve in the Nation's evolving health care system. The thoughts expressed grow out of my past work at Analytic Services, Inc. (ANSER) on the analysis of the cost-benefits of multiphasic health screening and my present work at ANSER on health benefit analysis in association with Drs. John Williamson and Charles Flagle on their Health Benefit Analysis Project (HBAP) at the Johns Hopkins University School of Hygiene and Public Health.

A major portion of health care in the United States is now provided under Medicare. Under present plans, organization of health service resources to provide care under Medicare funding will be accomplished through Health Maintenance Organizations (HMOs) established in each locality. Under other proposed plans, care would be extended to a major portion of the non-Medicare population through such HMOs. Because of the size of the public investment, operation of these HMOs must be closely monitored. Part of the monitoring function is evaluation, nationwide and in each HMO, of the quality of health care delivered under Medicare and other federally funded health plans. Evaluation requires the establishment of criteria against which performance can be assessed.

Systematic assessment of the quality of patient management and its outcome is most notable for its absence in most health care programs. Each physician dispensing care has his own criteria. In some cases, the criteria have been carefully and deliberately formulated; in others, more or less unconsciously evolved. In either case, they are based largely on the physician's own concept of (1) his knowledge of the state of the art of health care, (2) his relationship with and responsibility to his patient, and (3) the patient's need and resources. The physician applies these criteria as and when circumstances permit and usually subjectively. His knowledge and capability to administer care were measured formally by the medical school which trained him, the physicians who supervised him as an intern,

Harry E. Emlet, Jr., *Analytic Services, Inc., Falls Church, Va.*

This paper was read at the SAMS meeting by David Dittmet, Ph.D.

and to some degree, by the medical director of the organization in which he practices medicine if he is not among the vast majority in independent private practice. In most cases, neither his capability to administer care nor the quality of care he administers has been measured formally in any way since he was an intern. In situations where one physician supervises another, he normally assesses the other in pretty much the same manner as he assesses his own practice.

Some health research organizations and some individual physicians with a particular objective or research interest have systematically studied the outcome of the care they provide. Individual physicians usually do so in select areas of particular interest and on whatever population happens to be available. These investigations frequently yield valuable insights into care for special health problems and populations but leave major gaps in overall understanding of outcomes as related to generally accepted kinds and levels of care. Health research organizations have focused their efforts largely on the pathology of particular diseases or the development and refinement of particular care techniques and only rarely on the quality of health care, *per se,* of a population. These factors doubtless are major reasons why the art of assessing health care is still in a primitive state. No specific criteria for management and outcome of health care have been generally accepted, although from time to time, select groups have attempted to establish criteria for specific health problems and purposes.

However, most physicians, health service personnel and laymen would agree that the overall goals of health care should be to maintain or improve health, reduce impairment, extend life and thereby contribute to the preservation of economic viability and the quality of life. These goals then, at least, can become overall criteria for the outcome of health care if the extent to which they are attainable is known. Unfortunately, very little data exist as a basis for identifying expected outcomes for different levels of care. Also, generally agreed upon definitions of accepted levels of care for various health problems do not exist. Fortunately, work which we now have under way at ANSER and The Johns Hopkins University on health benefit analysis offers an interim means for obtaining agreed upon definitions of the outcomes of three levels of care: none, average and optimum. In the Health Benefit Analysis Project, these outcomes are estimated by persons identified by the medically informed community as the experts on specific health problems. Not only does the HBAP methodology assist in identifying outcomes, but it also aids in identifying the associated care and cost. It thus provides a uniquely appropriate tool for evaluating HMO programs of patient management and outcomes. It does this by providing a means for the medical community itself to establish outcome criteria based on the experience and knowledge of the experts on each health problem.

Initially, the criteria can be of a fairly general nature. A gross criterion could be the number of persons in the population at each of several major levels of impairment. More specific criteria could be the number of persons with a given health problem at each of the impairment levels. A set of health problems considered to be good indicators might be selected. In either case, the number expected with average care and with optimum care could be estimated. These two sets of values would then establish the boundaries of the acceptable range of performance.

Substantial latitude could exist in the selection of levels of impairment for which criteria are established. In HBAP we are now using six levels of impairment:

1. Well
2. Detectable
3. Symptomatic
4. Unable to work
5. Bedridden
6. Dead

Many other and more detailed indexes of impairment have been considered, but at the present stage of criteria development in health services, the simplicity of this set provides many advantages.

However, application of any criteria, regardless of how detailed, to the HMO population requires a means of assessing either the entire population or a random sample to determine health status. Initially, some fairly simple form of evaluation, such as a random sample poll by telephone or mail, could serve as a step in the right direction. However, more definitive means of assessment would soon be required. An acceptable means needs at least four attributes: it must be reliable, permit comparison of HMOs, be as independent as possible of the physician(s) who normally deliver care to the patient, and be low in cost. AMHT can have all of these attributes.

Reliability is concerned with the repeatability of the results. AMHT would be very much more reliable than polling of individuals and would be limited chiefly by the sensitivity and specificity of the tests.

Comparability (of sensitivity and specificity, particularly) is important to ensure that the evaluation is equitable among HMOs. The results of AMHT could be made comparable between HMOs through standardization of tests and test procedures and through cross calibration (calibration with common standards).

Independence of the assessment from the physician(s) who normally deliver care is important if maximum objectivity is to be achieved. AMHT would be independent because the physician(s) normally providing diagnosis and care would not be managing the AMHT laboratory.

Low cost is important to avoid undue diversion of resources from direct care. AMHT can be provided, based on experience at Kaiser and elsewhere, for less than $20 per person per examination. Annual screening of a population of 100,000 would cost less than $2 million − a cost of about 6% of the average annual expenditure per capita for health care today. If the sole purpose of the screening were HMO evaluation, only a fraction of the population − say 5% or less − would need to be sampled every two to four years. (This might mean that establishment of an AMHT facility for each individual HMO would not be feasible. Instead, centrally located or mobile AMHT facilities could service several HMOs, either as shared or separate contract operations.) Thus, the health appraisal as a basis for HMO evaluation could be provided at a cost of less than 25 to 50 cents per person in the population per year. If the screening were the regular annual health assessment performed as part of a preventive health maintenance program, the data would be available as a by-product of normal care.

The complete schedule of AMHT tests could vary somewhat from one HMO to another as long as each patient received certain basic tests in a standardized manner which would permit comparison among HMOs. If AMHT were used only for HMO evaluation, then a completely standard set of basic tests could be used.

A very attractive feature of an AMHT-based HMO evaluation procedure is that it inherently provides a means for improving the criteria. As the AMHT data accumulated from the many different participating HMOs, a more and more complete data base would become available for identifying health profiles for various populations. While estimation would continue to be required to establish criteria, the establishment of HMO evaluation criteria would be increasingly based on hard data produced by AMHT.

The evaluations could be used in two ways. First, the performance of the HMO could be rated on the basis of how closely the impairment status of the HMO population approaches that expected under optimum care. This rating could be a basis for providing dollar performance rewards and thus be an incentive for improved performance. Second, where impairment in the HMO population is significantly greater than that estimated by the experts for average care, a special investigation could be initiated to determine the cause. When cause for the discrepancy is established, corrective action, if needed, could be taken.

Corrective action could take various forms. It might, for example, initially be a recommendation to the HMO to improve its performance. If this did not produce results, the next action might be a warning that unless performance improved, the appropriate public agency would need to take corrective action. If there were still no satisfactory response, that agency could take more stringent measures − if necessary, revoking the HMOs charter. Various other forms of corrective action can be conceived. The possibility of such action would strongly motivate existing HMOs and their health services components to maintain high performance standards.

In summary, the magnitude of the Nation's resources that would be channeled under current plans through HMOs for health care, requires that the quality of care be monitored and evaluated. Means exist by which the experts within the medical community could establish initial criteria. AMHT could provide an effective and efficient means of generating the health status data which are needed for application of the evaluation criteria. The HMOs could then be evaluated by comparing the selected results from the AMHT with the estimated criteria, and an incentive system could be introduced to motivate the HMOs to maintain and improve the quality of health care.

Admitting Screening at Latter-Day Saints Hospital

T. Allan Pryor and Homer R. Warner

Routine screening of scheduled admissions at the Latter-Day Saints Hospital in Salt Lake City, Utah has been on-going since May 1968. Figure 1 depicts the floor plan of the present screening facility. Approximately 30% of all admissions to Latter Day Saints Hospital are processed through this facility. Patients classified as emergency are not admitted through the screening facility, but taken directly to their rooms. As a result, the population presently being processed is primarily scheduled surgical patients. A typical day's operation in the screening facility would amount to approximately 40 patients during the hours of 1:00 to 4:30 p.m., with a maximum flow of ten patients per hour. The facility is connected directly to a Control Data 3300 Computer, seven floors above, which is operated by the Intermountain Regional Medical Program in Salt Lake City.

The patient's first interface with the system is through a self-administered computer history. These history questions are written on a set of flip charts attached to an IBM Data Recorder. Figure 2 shows such a data recorder. As the patient reads through the set of questions, he responds to a positive answer by punching through a perforated IBM card which has been inserted in the Data Recorder. Rather than having a set time to complete this history, the patient is interrupted as is necessary for the performance of other screening procedures. At the completion of those tests he continues the history at the point where he left off. The patient's history, contained on the IBM card, and a second card, on which is punched the patient's name and identification number, are read by a small Hewlett-Packard card reader and processed by the computer. The positive responses to the questions are printed out immediately, using a Texas Instrument 30-character-per-second terminal.

The set of screening procedures performed on the patient can be divided into two classes. The first class is that set of procedures for which a report is printed upon completion of the tests and is available along with

---

T. Allan Pryor, Ph.D. *and* Homer R. Warner, M.D., Ph.D., *Latter-Day Saints Hospital, Salt Lake City, Utah.*

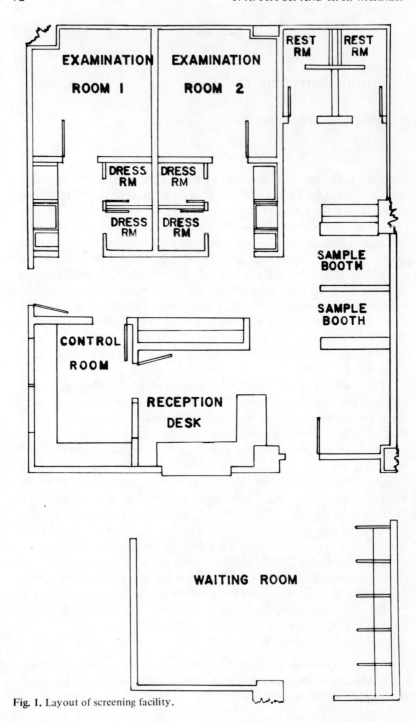

Fig. 1. Layout of screening facility.

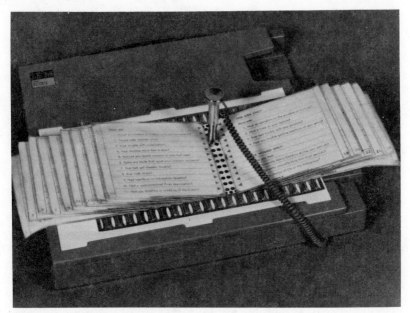

Fig. 2. Automated history recorder.

the patient history for review at the conclusion of the screen. These reports are taken with the patient and placed upon his chart as he arrives at his room, thus available for observation by the attending staff before workup of the patient. The second class of tests are those for which the results are not available on completion of the screen and are attached to the patient's chart approximately two to three hours following the performance of such tests.

Included in the Class 1 tests are the patient's vital statistics: age, sex, height, weight, blood pressure and temperature. Each of these is entered manually into the computer through a terminal with a numeric keyboard located in the multiphasic screening area. Three automated tests are also included in Class 1. One is an automated pulmonary function test administered directly on-line, giving the patient's total vital capacity, as well as the one-second expired volume. This test is repeated several times until the values are within normal range, or the patient has clearly performed a maximal test. The second test is an automated electrocardiogram in which the 12 standard leads are recorded, as well as the modified Frank lead ˎsystem. The vector X, Y, Z, leads are simultaneously transmitted to the computer for automatic interpretation and classification of both the waveform morphology and rhythm. A final automated test measures the patient's intraocular pressure and screens for glaucoma using a Marg-Mackay Tonometer. The Tonometer is also interfaced directly to the computer with the base line and trough of the intraocular pressure wave-form being extracted automatically and the pressure reported on-line to the technician. As mentioned above for these Class 1 tests, a report is immediately generated for the patient.

The Class 2 procedures are (1) the 12-channel automated chemistry determination, (2) a complete blood count, (3) urinalysis, and (4) a serological test for syphilis. The results of these tests are reported from the laboratory approximately two hours after receipt of the specimens from the patient. In the case of the chemistry determinations, the sample is read by the computer on-line from a Technicon SMA 12/60 and the report generated by the computer. The urinalysis and blood count results are entered manually into the system, using one of the computer terminals available in the laboratory area.

Another important function of the screening area is to initiate a medical record on the patient. This record is automatically generated on a magnetic disc as the vital statistics from the patient are entered into the system. All results from the screening tests are added to the record. During the patient's stay the record will be continually updated with other measurements from different areas within the hospital. At discharge the record is completed with the addition of discharge diagnostic information and then transferred from active file on disc to magnetic tape for long-term storage, medical audit function, research and for review if the patient is re-admitted.

Not only are the test results stored on discs by patient, but these results are also subjected to analysis by a series of logical and arithmetic statements which are stored on discs. These statements represent the currently accepted criteria for medical decisions such as the presence of a "moderate respiratory problem due to airway obstruction." When such a decision has been made, a corresponding bit in the patient's record is set which allows inquiry or report programs to recognize the presence of this condition without having to repeat the original sequence of logical manifestations. Also, other decision making later in the patient's stay may make reference to those bits, e.g., the diagnosis of aortic insufficiency at heart catheterization depends on prior decisions made in screening by the electrocardiographic analysis program which also sets diagnostic bits, and the decision to put in a pacemaker in a patient who develops an A-V block while being monitored in the coronary care unit may depend on the prior diagnosis of anterior myocardial infarction by the ECG morphology program. Thus, it can be seen that the screening data are the basis for an automated problem-oriented patient record designed to facilitate not only the medical audit, but also on-line decision making within the hospital.

In evaluating the performance of the screening facility, two questions were asked:

1. What is the percent of abnormals resulting from the various screening procedures?
2. Of what value is this information to the clinician?

In answering the first question, statistics were generated from approximately 4500 patients with the following results being obtained. In 29% of the patients some abnormality was detected in the ECG morphology. A further breakdown of the morphological analysis showed that in 15% of the cases an abnormality was present in the QRS complex, and in 23% of the cases an abnormality was present in the ST segment or T wave. ECG rhythm abnormalities were measured in 11% of the cases. To answer the second question, selected patients were reviewed to determine physician follow-up. Follow-up was defined for the purpose of this study as "any evidence found in the chart indicating acknowledgement of the abnormality." This included repeated tests, consultation, alteration of patient schedule, comments on doctors' notes, etc. In 100% of the cases where the patient had been admitted for a cardiovascular problem, the abnormal ECG was mentioned in the physician's write-up and followed up. However, in those cases where cardiovascular disease was not his chief complaint, only 25% of the charts indicated some type of follow-up.

In reviewing the spirometry results, it was found that 17% of the patients had a forced vital capacity less than 80% of predicted and 23% of the patients had a one-second volume less than 80% of predicted. Again, in all instances where the respiratory problem was the patient's chief complaint, follow-up was mentioned by the clinician. However, only 20% of the abnormalities were mentioned when a respiratory problem was not the chief complaint of that patient.

Table 1 gives the percentage of abnormal tests for each of the 12 chemistry determinations measured by the SMA 12. It is noted here that

TABLE 1. Percentage of Abnormal Chemistry Tests

Cholesterol	11%
Calcium	22%
Phosphorus	17%
Bilirubin	12%
Albumin	25%
Total Protein	7%
Uric Acid	26%
BUN	17%
Glucose	43%
LDH	12%
Alkaline Phosphatase	13%
SGOT	8%

the high percentage (43%) of abnormal glucose probably results from the fact that the patients were not requested to enter the hospital in a fasting state. Eighty-six percent (86%) of the patients had at least one abnormal chemistry determination. If the glucose test is excluded, the percent of abnormals drops only to 78%. As has been mentioned by other investigators, the clinical significance of these isolated abnormal chemical results is still not known. It is noted here, however, that if the tests were assumed independent, one would expect 45% of the patients to have at least one abnormality. This is true using the 5% significance level. For approximately 60% of the abnormalities, evidence was found in the chart to indicate evaluation by the physician.

At the time of this study, written histories by the attending physician were also required by the hospital in conjunction with the computer history. An evaluation was undertaken to study the usefulness of the computer history in reporting information of value to the doctor. This was accomplished by comparing the computer history with the doctor's history. The histories were broken into two categories.— those for medical patients and those for surgical patients. For medical patients, 79% of the "yes" responses to the computer history were also mentioned within the doctor's history, whereas 65% of the "yes" responses were mentioned by the doctors of the surgical patient. For 16% of the medical patients, the chief complaint was not mentioned in the computer history; and for 18% of the surgical patients, the chief complaint was not mentioned in the computer history. In reviewing these cases, it was found that some of the patients had psychological problems and did not complete an accurate history, several of the patients were old and confused by the questionnaire, and for a number of the cases the set of questions in the computer history did not include the chief complaint (e.g., a surgical patient with a lymph node enlargement).

Perhaps the most striking statistic in this evaluation was the percentage of patients for which the computer history drew to the attention of the physician an unknown secondary problem. This was found in 19% of the medical patients and in 10% of the surgical patients. In general, the specific differences between the two histories were found in reviewing family history. Here, the computer tended to be more detailed in its questionnaire set, whereas the doctors were more thorough in the review of systems and, in particular, in evaluating the chief complaint for which the patient was being admitted to the hospital. Much more information corresponding to secondary problems was detailed by the computer history than was found in the history compiled by the doctors.

In continuing this project, evaluation of the procedures is the key. New tests must be reviewed both for their feasibility for integration into the present system, and their justification from the point of view of clinical information before inclusion in the screening system. Old tests need to be continually reviewed and upgraded.

This work was supported by a grant through the Intermountain Regional Medical Program.

An AMHT Program: Its Use in the Care
of the Sick and Evaluation of the Asymptomatic

Malcolm Schwartz

The United States Public Health Service; the Department of Health, Education and Welfare; and our state Regional Medical Program have inspected and reviewed our program on multiple occasions. Referral to our center from these sources has come about following patient request for services such as we provide.

Our study suggests that health performance should be measured in all people whose longevity, productivity and state of well-being would be threatened if it were not done. Disease detection should be limited to those who, uninterrupted in the asymptomatic phase, would cause harm to the community through spread or higher treatment cost. Eligible for early detection would be diseases whose progression could be aborted, delayed or attenuated in ability to produce pain, to disable or to shorten lifespan.

In the care of the sick, it was noted that hospital-associated income has decreased, as has bed utilization. The level of nursing care is higher in currently admitted patients, and laboratory testing is more sophisticated. There is a greater dependence on our non-hospital-affiliated, out-patient center because of the ease and lower cost of data acquisition. Our hospital does not have automated facilities other than for blood testing. The fee is higher than independent laboratories. The facility chosen by the physician is usually dictated by qualifying circumstances of payment and ease of obtaining information (if treatment can be given on an out-patient basis).

I have functioned in the past two years in a dual role. The first is that of a family doctor and the second as the president of a for-profit company. We develop automated and manual systems for clinical applications. The purpose of these systems is to increase physician productivity while stimulating a measurably superior level of patient care. The development of a for-profit company was stimulated by our inability to get government funds for the program. It was felt that a community

---

Malcolm Schwartz, M.D., *President, Automated Screening Centers, Inc., Des Plaines, Ill.*

physician's needs and experience were unique and worth considering. This is in light of his high level of productivity (measured in hours and number of patients seen per day). If his availability could be enhanced, other formats of health care delivery would benefit as well.

This presentation deals with my experience in utilizing automated multiphasic health testing and multiple diagnostic-assisting computer programs in the care of the sick, and in evaluation of asymptomatic population.

Our AMHT unit is in a 440-square-foot building which houses a pharmacy and physicians' offices, representing three specialties and general practice. The laboratory and x-ray are independent. The screening center contracts the services of these two facilities. It occupies 475 square feet and shares the common building waiting room. During the hours of AMHT operation, the x-ray facility limits its activities to its demands.

The AMHT unit is divided into four areas. The first is for patient registration. This is also the site of data processing. The second room contains two terminals for self-administered patient histories. The third room is for audio-visual testing, which is patient administered. The fourth room is for additional physiologic data collected by a registered nurse. This includes electrocardiography, tonometry and pulmonary function. The ECG is on-line for real time analysis. All other data is direct terminal entry from sensors to audio tape. Laboratory studies and x-ray reports are hand entered. The patient usually has the hands-on portion of the examination performed immediately following completion of testing. The patient history and physiological data, including ECG, is available at that time.

The complex has been used as a physician's assistant. It has more than doubled the number of physical examinations that I could perform in the course of the office day. It has allowed a 25% increase in the total number of patients seen. The program is a total-care, fee-for-service one, under the direction of a family physician. Other than general patient load, patients are referred from a methadone program and a poly-drug abuse program. Other sources of referral include the U.S. Public Health Service; Regional Medical Programs; Health, Education and Welfare; the American Cancer Society; industry; insurance companies and other physicians.

The patient benefits by remaining actively employed, in many cases, as well as being at home with his family. The health insurance carrier or purchaser of the service saves the cost of room and board.

With the availability of computer diagnostic-assisting programs in Electrocardiography, Internal Medicine and Pediatrics, the weakest link is my ability to acquire valid data from the hands-on portion of the physical examination. I believe postgraduate education should stress skills, tools and modes of data acquisition. Each patient experience will then be postgraduate training with complete and current information. The physician will not have to take time from care of the sick to seek information which is soon forgotten and poorly reinforced.

We are still a major underutilized resource in the community. Proper utilization will require the support of those who control the patient's income and the health insurance carrier in motivating the community to demand total-care programs dependent on quality economies for their success.

The above comments are based on my first year's experience with the asymptomatic, or solicited, patient and the routine patient load of a family practitioner. The presentation must be considered an initial impression, as the data is still in the stage of analysis.

The site of the program was an upper-middle-class community, with high school graduation as the lower level of adult educational attainment. We would be considered a medically affluent community because of our physician-to-patient ratio, as well as in the availability of medical facilities.

A Health Testing Concept: Simple-By-Design

William R. Duff and Harry S. Lipscomb

Introduction

As a nation, U.S. citizens spent 7% of the Gross National Product, or $70 billion, on health care in 1970.[1] Both relatively and absolutely, this is more than any other nation in the world has invested in the treatment of disease. In return for this outlay, a significant number of Americans received superb care when suffering with life-threatening illness. For these individuals we have used our technology and personnel in an effective fashion. For many in our nation, however, the promise of our technology has remained unfulfilled and the cost of entry has prevented easy access early in the course of illness. Virtually no mechanisms exist for frequent, regular, inexpensive health checkups and simple reassurance concerning health status. In short, Americans must be sick to seek health care and must be prepared to pay for it. For the poor and near-poor, the illness must be of catastrophic dimensions.

Comprehensive health care for the future should stress preventive health; provide easy, low-cost entry; and insure a continuum of care for all people. Separate systems for rich and poor are not the answer. If costs for health care are to be lowered in this country, early ambulatory health care must be emphasized.

One of the most promising ideas in this regard has been the concept of a periodic general health examination in which a search is made for health as well as disease, and in which the patient is examined *out of the hospital*. The examination should encompass an investigation of the whole person, including all major organ-systems, and should search generically for disease rather than concentrate upon a single disease, such as diabetes, cancer, or heart disease. Importantly, such an examination should be viewed as but the first step in the total sequence of comprehensive health care.

New Health Care Systems

The past 20 years have seen an increasing interest in health testing systems for diagnostic and predictive purposes, variously termed multi-

William R. Duff, Ph.D. *and* Harry S. Lipscomb, M.D., *Xerox Center for Health Care Research, Baylor College of Medicine, Texas Medical Center, Houston, Tex.*

phasic screening, automated multiphasic health testing, health maintenance examinations, etc. All possess basic conceptual similarities: the
ultimate goal being to provide, medically and economically, more effective
health surveillance for large populations. In most instances the testing
procedures are intended to be of a screening nature (i.e., distinguish the
early sick from the basically well).

General trends of existing programs have been toward technological
sophistication. Computers and automated equipment have been used
extensively to perform and calculate individual test procedures as well as
to process the total set of data for presentation to a physician. Computers
and automated equipment can reduce operating costs in certain applications but there are many instances where computer usage cannot be
economically justified. Present testing systems make frequent use of
detailed, automated medical histories. A patient interfaces with a
computer terminal and responds to a branched set of medical questions.
The procedure frequently takes 30 to 60 minutes of a patient's time. In
many cases a physician, when presented with the history summary, will
repeat questions and perform his individual style of free-form branching. It
would seem that a quicker, less expensive method could be found to direct
a physician to areas needing his attention and further questioning.

The biochemical procedures performed on blood and urine follow
similar approaches. Costly automated systems are used to measure
biochemical parameters of questionable yield.[2]

Some of the more recent automated multiphasic health testing systems
appear to be working for certain fixed populations (industrial, military or
group medical practices), yet even here more conclusive evaluations are
needed.[3] Their complexity, cost and demand for mass patient flow have
delayed their adoption and it appears that the concepts of existing
programs have failed to exert a significant national impact upon the cost
and availability of quality health care for all people.

A SIMPLE-BY-DESIGN Health Testing Concept

Based upon studies at the Xerox Center for Health Care Research in
Houston, a departure has been made from the complexities and expense of
conventional screening programs. We have developed a concept for health
testing which has as its primary constraint that such systems be
simple-by-design. Given this criterion, such systems must be inexpensive;
health care personnel must be used as effectively as possible; and the
system must be sufficiently adaptable to insure wide, effective application.
Unless computers or automated techniques can be shown to be relevant
and economical, they should not be used. Testing procedures should be
vital to the diagnosis of disease or the identification of health and,

thereby, useful to both patient and physician. A health testing system which is simple-by-design, flexible, low in cost, and which uses limited health manpower more effectively might, in truth, see early widespread adoption into comprehensive, ambulatory health care programs throughout the nation.

It has been reasoned that a prime factor in the high costs of health care has been the unwillingness of private health insurance carriers to fund out-patient diagnostic procedures, thus forcing excessive and inappropriate use of our hospitals. Indeed, of the $70 billion outlay, at least 38% has gone for hospital costs.[4] We believe, however, that when the real issues are examined, it will be found that insurance companies have not funded ambulatory health care because we have lacked an orderly, systematic, low-cost, out-patient care system.

A Research Model

The first prototype of a system to meet the above concepts has been operational as a research model at Baylor College of Medicine for the past six months. Historical, biochemical and physiological measurements are obtained, processed and presented to the physician (or health manager) for his review. At present, the procedure requires approximately 30 minutes. The patient then meets with a physician to discuss the results of the testing. The facility is operated by health technicians trained to perform specific sets of functions.

The Baylor facility consists of only two patient stations. At the first station basic reception and identification take place, a history is taken and blood and urine samples are obtained. The patient then goes to the second test station where multiple physiological measurements are made with the patient in a comfortable, relaxed position. During this interval a manual analysis of blood and urine is performed. A manual information-management system has been developed to allow effective collection and presentation of data. This research model can be modified easily and applied diversely: various facilities, e.g., neighborhood health centers, mobile units, hospitals and doctors' offices; various populations, e.g., school children, veterans and disadvantaged; various purposes, e.g., predictive, diagnostic and presurgical.

The history is specifically designed to identify abnormality of function and is being developed to provide the physician with key words that will quickly direct his attention to a potential problem area. The health technician is taught to ask categorical questions in an easy, flexible manner, and the patient is asked to respond in simple affirmative or negative answers. The present history consists of 20 questions and is administered in approximately four minutes. While not as detailed as conventional 200-400 question histories, it is intended that this short questioning would reveal almost all problems detected by a longer history. The concept can be seen from one of the questions: "Do you have pain anywhere?" No other "pain" questions are asked. If a person says "yes" to this question from the health technician, the physician can later branch quickly to the important detailed questions concerning location, duration, quality, intensity or relief. Furthermore, experience with existing self-administered detailed questions of pain in every body area, with branched subsets in positive areas, results in a print-out to which the typical physician *still* exercises his cardinal option: " . . . tell me about it." This observation has led us to search for a simple history questionnaire that excludes those branched questions which the physician does, in fact, repeat.

Presently, a mix of several serological, hemotological, bacteriological and biochemical procedures on blood and urine is being performed. A totally manual system of pertinent measurements is being developed into a small system allowing the health technician to perform the measurements on-line in approximately ten minutes. Procedures chosen for such a system must depend upon the specific clinical application.

A carefully selected set of measurements is taken at the physiological test station. Each procedure (as with each historical and laboratory parameter) is under scrutiny for relevance and effectiveness. Measurements are taken by the technician, using instruments housed in a console around the patient. Presently, all measurements are taken in approximately 18 minutes, including height, weight, spirometry (FEV_1, FVC, FEV_1/FVC and ratios to predicted values), vision (distance, near point, color, depth perception and phoria), audiometry, blood pressure, oral temperature and electrocardiogram (6 leads). As an example of the research directions, a project is underway to replace the electrocardiogram (currently read by a physician) with an inexpensive ECG computer, designed to indicate simply that the patient does or does not require a detailed electrocardiogram.

While the research population studied has had routine chest x-rays, the importance of routine x-rays for inclusion in a simple-by-design health testing system must ultimately be determined by specific clinical needs and the population being screened. Routine mass chest x-ray studies of all age groups have not had a significant yield.[5]

The model developed and operated in Houston meets our boundary conditions in some cases and falls short in others. The fact that over 40 separate parameters can be obtained in less than 30 minutes without the use of automation or computers speaks for the simple and expeditious nature of the system. This has been accomplished by more effective use of allied health personnel and methodology in a sharply limited geographic area. Clothing is not removed and patients are not shuttled from one area to another. There is no waiting and the time saved for the patient encourages enthusiastic participation.

The brief history has proven highly useful in quickly focusing upon the patient's problems. Nutritional, social and behavioral areas are currently being studied for simple, alerting answers which the physician may explore in depth.

The goal of relevance for all testing procedures has been only partially fulfilled and constitutes the major research thrust for the future. It appears that more simple, high-yield testing procedures in physiology and biochemistry are needed. Routine hearing testing has had questionable usefulness. In keeping with the need for flexibility, however, hearing testing is retained for populations such as school-age children where early correction of hearing problems is important. Routine studies of bacteria in urine, vision testing and pulmonary and cardiovascular testing have uncovered significant problems in an ostensibly "well" population, and this may rise sharply when one screens the aged and the disadvantaged.

The multiple biochemical measurements routinely performed on blood have had a relatively low yield, and it is concluded that within the concept developed here, existing, highly quantitative tests should be made simpler and provide only high, low or normal answers. Kinetic measurements of key rate-limiting steps in metabolism using simple biochemical measurements are being investigated.

A hidden benefit has been the encouragement of the physician to spend more time with his patient and less time in the search for data. Additionally, the patient's problems can be reviewed in the framework of his total life style, rather than as isolated problems. Another benefit of incalculable value has been the reassurance that such a comprehensive examination provides the patient when all tests are normal. This tends to provide a positive reinforcement to health education and the concept of preventive health maintenance among patients and their families.

The health technicians are taught to rotate in their roles so that levels of efficiency are maintained through variety. One of the authors has served a dual role, both as health technician and as physician-health manager. A technician is being taught to perform and record a rather detailed physical examination without exercising judgmental decisions.

It is critical to recognize that in all of this, from history, laboratory testing and the physiological test battery, the physician retains all options. The historian is, in fact, encouraged to record minimally positive responses, allowing the physician to exercise his own judgment as to significance.

Health testing as described here constitutes only one step in the complex process of comprehensive health care, which begins with patient awareness of the importance of seeking help. Entry, testing, diagnosis, treatment, referral and follow-up care must be accomplished with dignity, at low cost and with easy access for everyone. This must be done earlier, before disease is advanced, if potential savings in money, time and human life are to be realized. The estimated basic cost for setting up such a testing system in clinics, doctors' offices or hospitals should not exceed $15,000, and the operating cost per patient should be between $10 and $20. Based upon limited observations, but bolstered by recognition of need for broader health education and saving of time for physician and patient, the economics of the concept described here offers a simple first approach to the solution of a critical national problem.

References

1. President Richard M. Nixon: Health message to the Congress of the United States, Feb. 18, 1971.
2. Automated multiphasic health testing in the seventies. *Westchester Medical Society*, June 14, 1970, p. 92.
3. Thorner, R. M.: Whither multiphasic screening? *New Eng. J. Med.*, 280:1037-1042, 1969.
4. Faltermayer, E. K.: Better care at less cost without miracles. *Fortune*, 80, Jan. 1970.
5. Tizes, R. and Tizes, C. W.: Decline in statewide mobile x-ray programs to detect tuberculosis. *Public Health Rep.*, 85:901-904, 1970.

Entry Point Linkages to Comprehensive Health Services

Melvyn Greberman

One of the major areas of concern of health planners at the present time is how patients enter health care systems.

Consider first the classical mechanism by which patients enter the health care system in this country. Some important features are:

1. The patient enters the system through his own awareness of the problem and desire for relief.
2. He goes where he thinks he can be helped, based on his own limited personal experience and that of his peers.
3. After seeing a physician, the patient may return to the population or receive further care on an out-patient or in-patient basis.
4. After the problem is resolved, the patient returns to the population.
5. When the next crisis arises, he may or may not see the same physician.

Although this description is to some degree simplistic, it is, unfortunately, somewhat accurate.

We are all aware of the problems associated with this system and have seen examples to a varying degree:

1. The patient who does not obtain help until his problem is far advanced because of lack of awareness of the seriousness of the situation, because of lack of knowledge of where to seek health care, or because of inaccessibility of services.
2. The patient who is treated for a presenting complaint but not for some more serious problem because the physician lacks more complete knowledge of his patient's health status.
3. The patient who is evaluated without regard to important social or environmental factors.
4. The patient who does not follow the physician's instructions because he does not understand them or realize the significance of his own problems.

Melvyn Greberman, M.S., M.D., M.P.H., *Health Services Research, U.S. Public Health Service Hospital, Baltimore, Md.*

5. The physician who is too busy or simply unable to determine whether his patient has followed his advice or obtained additional services.

We could list several more examples, but these will serve as adequate background for the discussion to follow.

Certainly more and more attention is being focused on the problems of health services accessibility and continuity and comprehensiveness of health care. We will review some of the current concepts and programs being considered.

Primary Care

One of the most frequently discussed ideas is that of primary care. Primary care "describes a range of services adequate for meeting the great majority of daily personal health needs."[1] It is most often used by patients who are ambulatory and includes the "need for preventive health maintenance and for the evaluation and management on a continuing basis of general discomfort, early complaints, symptoms, problems and chronic intractable aspects of disease."

Once care has been sought, the primary care program should assure continuity of all care the patient may subsequently need. It does not itself provide comprehensive health services, but serves as "the entry and continuity point for comprehensive care."[1] The primary care program must make sure that ready access to more specialized and intensive care is available to patients of the program.

As described in "A Conceptual Model of Organized Primary Care and Comprehensive Community Health Services,"[1] the *sine qua non* of organized primary care is the primary care team. This team must provide three essential services: primary medical care, nursing care, and health outreach and social advocacy.

Among providers of primary medical care are family practice physicians, internists, pediatricians, physician assistants, nurse practitioners and pediatric associates. Nursing care may be provided by registered nurses, public health nurses, visiting nurses, licensed practical nurses, nurse's aides and home health aides.

"Health outreach refers to work in the community of an informational nature – both giving information to and collecting it from individual persons – most often in the context of follow-up after medical care. Social advocacy refers to the service of intervening for individuals who need help in securing access to a health or social service."[1] Health outreach and social advocacy are provided by social workers, public health nurses, family health workers, community health aides and patient advocates.

Depending on the needs of the population served, the primary care program will have on-site services or provide arrangements for other medical services, such as obstetrical and dental care and services that support the program, such as x-ray and pharmacy.

As part of being the key element in a comprehensive community health services program, an organized primary care program should provide services to the community at large. Among these are community organization and citizen participation, control measures for communicable and environmental risk-related diseases, environmental improvement activities, health education and promotional activities and health-related legal services.

Health Care Personnel

We will now investigate some ways in which new types of health personnel are being used to improve entry point linkages to health services.

In 1962, Congress passed the Migrant Health Act to make it possible for interested public or private agencies or organizations to provide health services for migratory farmworkers and their families. "As part of these services, local project sponsors were among the first professional groups in this country to recruit and employ persons who represented the migratory workers themselves. The indigenous workers, or health aides as they were usually called, were employed to bridge the cultural gap between the migrants and the professional staff, to improve communications between these groups, and to help deliver health services more effectively to migrant workers and their families."[2]

In addition to freeing professionals so that they could more fully use their specialized training and competence, health aides have helped "overcome barriers of cultural differences, professional status, communication difficulties, lack of motivation and understanding, and other difficulties that have interfered with providing health services."[2]

Health aides thus act as a bridge between the health agency and community and provide an entirely new linkage for the provision of health services. Some of their activities include identifying health interests and problems among migrants, casefinding, determining whether the physician's instructions are understood and followed, providing transportation to health services, orienting newly arrived families to the health services available, teaching people simple health practices, babysitting with children while parents obtain service and helping to find food, clothing, shelter and employment for those in need.

We see another example of innovative entry linkage in a project funded under Section 314(e) of the Public Health Service Act. Located in Elkins,

West Virginia, the Family Health Service administers a program of comprehensive health services for residents of Randolph County. Staffed by professional personnel and family health workers who are community residents trained locally in a special program, the Service provides "direct social outreach and home health services while referring patients needing medical care to cooperating practitioners and institutions of the patient's choice."[3]

The scope of the use of nonprofessionals in some health areas is evident in a study of 185 demonstration projects involving the use of nonprofessional workers in mental health service roles. In addition to providing service in various therapeutic settings and community adjustment problems, the nonprofessionals were heavily involved in entry linkage concerns such as casefinding and facilitation of access to project services. "Close to 90% of respondents surveyed indicated that their projects could not have functioned without the utilization of the nonprofessional group."[4]

Summary

To summarize, we have investigated the classical mechanisms by which patients enter the health care system in this country and certain problems associated with lack of patient sophistication, inaccessibility of services and lack of continuity and comprehensiveness. We have explored the concept of primary care programs and the key role they play as an entry point to health care services and as providers of continuity in care. We also noted some of the newer roles these programs may play in health care.

We then studied some programs in which new types of health personnel are providing more effective linkage between the population and health services to lessen the difficulties associated with cultural differences, problems in communication and lack of accessibility.

References

1. *A Conceptual Model of Organized Primary Care and Comprehensive Community Health Services,* P.H.S. Publication No. 2024. U.S. Department of Health, Education and Welfare, Division of Health Care Services, 1970.
2. Hoff, W.: *The Use of Health Aides in Migrant Health Projects,* Rockville, Md., U.S. Department of Health, Education and Welfare, Division of Health Care Services, 1970.
3. *A Directory of Selected Community Health Services Funded Under Section 314(e) of the Public Health Service Act,* Rockville, Md., U.S. Department of Health, Education and Welfare, Division of Health Care Services, 1970.
4. Sobey, F.: *Non-professional Personnel in Mental Health Programs: A Summary Report,* National Clearinghouse for Mental Health Information Publication No. 5028. Chevy Chase, Md., U.S. Department of Health, Education and Welfare, Health Services and Mental Health Administration, 1970.

Problems Associated With the
Automated Physician's Assistant

Alan H. Purdy

In the early months of 1970, a group of eight projects of the Missouri Regional Medical Programs — located at the University of Missouri, Columbia, Missouri — banded together under the heading of Advanced Technical Projects, later to be called the Automated Physician's Assistant. These groups were:

1. Automated Patient History, which had developed an audio-visual history;
2. Biomedical Engineering, which had developed physiological transduction apparatus;
3. Biochemical Screening, which had in operation an SMA 4, SMA 12 and other laboratory apparatus;
4. Computer Data Evaluation, which had been involved in experimental programs with several of the eight groups;
5. Electrocardiogram, which had developed a series of field stations using the Caceres program;
6. Computerized Library Service, which had developed an automated retrieval system using a Mosler 410 in conjunction with an IBM 360-50 computer;
7. Operations Research, which had developed operation plans for several screening systems, and finally;
8. Computerized Radiology, which had developed a method of automated reporting and diagnosis.

The Automated Physician's Assistant was directed to take its activities into the field with the objective of increasing health care delivery in rural areas. This was to be done by increasing the scope and sophistication of medical tests; decreasing the workload of the physician by cutting down the paperwork which currently consumes 10%-20% of his time; and encouraging the entrance of physicians into rural practice by ending their medical isolation, linking them to a modern medical center.

Alan H. Purdy, Ph.D., *Deputy Associate Director for Washington Operations, National Institute for Occupational Safety and Health, Department of Health, Education and Welfare, Rockville, Md.*

Our group was fortunate in finding an enthusiastic and cooperative physician, Billie Jack Bass, whose solo clinic at Salem, Missouri, was located 135 miles away over winding country roads. Fortunately, we had several pilots and airplanes in the group and this greatly facilitated services and conferences.

Salem is a small town of about 3900. The phone lines linking the Bass Clinic to the University of Missouri computers are approximately 225 miles long and involve three different telephone companies. Two of the lines are C-2 conditioned lines and the third is a WATS. Figure 1 is a simplified diagram of the communications network with the services listed.

The EKG is automated and can be either "on-line" or batched. The history is always on-line. As can be seen in Figure 1, the x-ray, blood chemistry, and hematology are carried by courier. All remaining information is entered into the system using an IBM 2260 CRT terminal or facsimile.

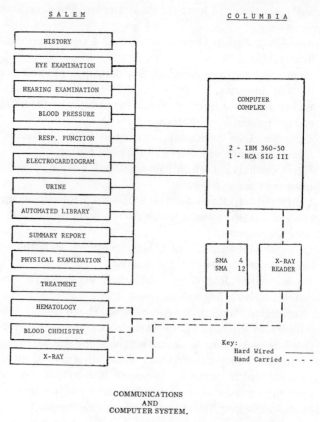

COMMUNICATIONS
AND
COMPUTER SYSTEM.

Figure 1.

The summary report is issued from the main computer to a high speed printer in the Clinic.

The original audio-visual automated patient history used an IMB 1050, Uher tape recorder and Kodak projector. We found, however, that patients and nurses preferred to use the automated history on the IBM 2260 CRT because of its greater speed and dependability.

The vision test remains to be automated because we found no commercial automated apparatus that would meet FAA standards, and we could not do this job ourselves.

The automatic hearing test uses a modified Tracore ARJ-4 with A/D conversion and digital readout added by Bioengineering.

The automatic blood pressure machine is an Air Shields Monitor with A/D conversion and digital readout added.

The respiratory function tester was manufactured by National Cylinder Gas, with A/D conversion and digital readout added.

The automatic EKG cart was designed and built in-house, with associated Burdick components. This unit uses the RCA Sigma III computer.

The computerized library uses a Mosler 410 linked to an IBM 360-50.

The facsimile machines are unmodified Grafic Science units.

The IBM 2260 CRT terminal handles the bulk of the data. This machine is also used to enter radiology data reports on diagnosis.

The blood chemistry and hematology are processed by an SMA 12 and SMA 4.

A number of good results have come from this project, not the least of which is that automated health care delivery has captured the attention of the press.

We also find that patients are generally pleased with the system and feel they are receiving exceptional care. Medical personnel, with a small amount of formal training, show the ability to operate the system. The physician is no longer isolated from a modern medical center and an overall improvement in quality of health care occurs because the summary report is a unified and thorough examination of the patient.

However, there are flaws in the system. As a single isolated system, it is far too expensive. A significant amount of data has been lost due to error in the computer system. Telephone lines between various parts of the system have not been entirely dependable. Some commercial and modified pieces of equipment have failed; extra personnel are required to operate the system because, at its present level of development, it consumes more time than it saves.

A number of changes are necessary to improve this system:

1. Lower cost by using the latest types of communication methods, telephone or otherwise.

2. Reduce cost by linking more physicians' offices to the computer;
3. Provide automatic hard copy of test entries at the physician's office;
4. Handle patient billing procedures;
5. Simplify the operation of medical instrumentation; and
6. Probably most important, automate the data interface between the test and the computer.

A new system has been designed to alleviate the shortcomings, but as yet we have not been successful in financing it.

Development of the Automated Physician's Assistant

Owen W. Miller, Gayle E. Adams, Earl M. Simmons, Jr.
and B. J. Bass

Mission of the Missouri Regional Medical Program

Medical science has made dramatic advances in establishing new knowledge for improved health care as well as developing new techniques for the delivery of health care.

The Missouri Regional Medical Program (MoRMP) began its activities in July 1966. MoRMP serves most of the state of Missouri with headquarters in Columbia, Missouri. It began funding operational projects in April 1967, the goals of these programs being twofold: (a) to improve access to the health delivery system for persons needing service and (b) to improve access to health information for persons providing services.

Advanced Technology Project

Eight of the initial projects were requested to combine their efforts, if possible, into a single project and to test, if possible, the results of their efforts in a private practicing physician's office for a field test evaluation. In July 1970 these eight separately funded projects merged, calling their effort the Advanced Technology Project (ATP).

These eight projects, each with a project director and funds to carry out each of their identified goals, were organized into a loose structure headed by an executive secretary. The University-wide administration brought together the resources of the School of Medicine and the College of Engineering through the Coordinator of the MoRMP and the Director of Operations of the MoRMP to form the Advanced Technology Project

Owen W. Miller, Sc.D. *Associate Professor, Department of Industrial Medicine;* Gayle E. Adams, Ph.D., *Professor, Department of Electrical Engineering; and* Earl M. Simmons, Jr., M.D., *Associate Professor, Department of Surgery, University of Missouri, Columbia, Mo.; and* B. J. Bass, M. D., *Private Practitioner, Salem, Mo.*

(ATP). Figure 1 lists the personnel who were initially involved in the ATP effort and shows the organizational structure.

The first six months of the ATP effort were spent developing a prototype of an integrated system which incorporated the products of each of the eight separately funded projects. The engineering projects served as the cohesive factor ("glue") to integrate the services developed by each of the separate projects. The prototype is, in effect, a comprehensive medical information system utilizing a computer to obtain, analyze, store and retrieve patient data.

The next step was to find a physician who would agree to be the initial field test site. Dr. B. J. Bass of Salem, Missouri, agreed to provide this test site.

The ATP, as illustrated in Figure 2, has succeeded in combining several types of expertise and focusing upon the objective of creating a system which will aid the physician. This system, which consists of computing equipment, communication lines, medical equipment and professional services has been called "The Automated Physician's Assistant."

Automated Physician's Assistant (APA)

The objective of this field demonstration project is to determine whether a sophisticated, advanced technology system can be installed, operated and effectively utilized in the private, rural physician's office. To date this system, presently the only one of its kind, has indicated that it has the potential to exert a significant influence on the delivery of health care. Allied health personnel, with a minimum of formal training, have demonstrated the required interest and ability needed to operate such a system, which, in effect, extends the physician's capabilities and will tend to lower medical costs while making a greater amount of medical information available to the physician. The physician, recognizing that this prototype does not represent an ideal system, has willingly given many hours to the modifications needed to make it a more effective tool for the delivery of health care. If such a system can be made widely available, it will surely attract young physicians to practice in rural areas, where, although they are vitally needed, the incentive for selecting such locations is lacking.

Figure 3 shows the categories of information which are presently included in the Automated Physician's Assistant. Information within some or all of these categories, as directed by the physician, is obtained about each patient during his visit to the physician's office. All of the information about each patient is stored in a computer file from which a summary report can be extracted in a form that is convenient to the

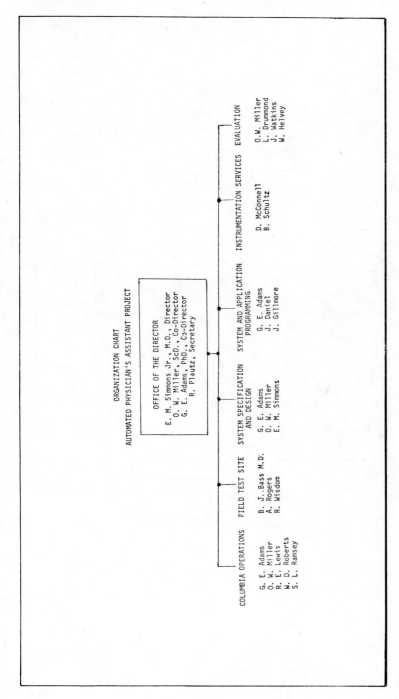

Figure 1.

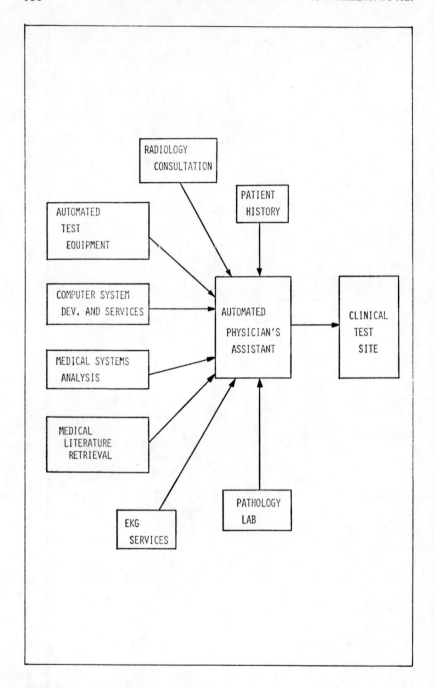

Figure 2.

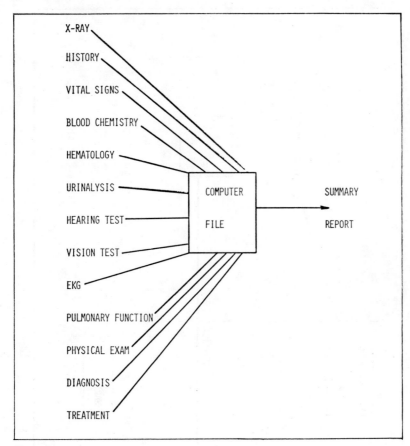

Figure 3.

physician. The physician is interested in the picture of the patient's health as painted by the complete report.

Figure 4 indicates that the computer file and the physician's office are connected by telephone lines, demonstrating that the APA can be used in locations remote from computer facilities. The figure also indicates that other means of communication such as courier can be used to transport blood samples and x-ray film to specialized consulting laboratories which in turn can enter the pertinent medical information in the computer file. The physician can then look to the one central source for his information about the patient.

Figure 5 illustrates the history obtained as the result of the patient answering questions displayed on either the typewriter-like or TV-like terminal. Using either device, questions are asked wherein the patient

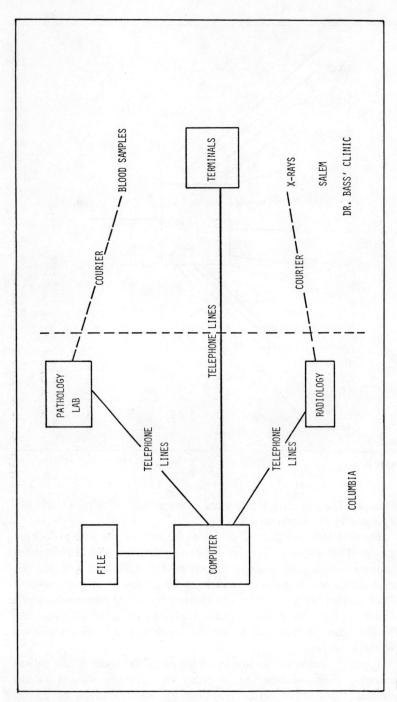

Figure 4.

```
ATP REPORT 01/18/71 10:05  0001724                          HISTORY
        63  YEAR OLD
_____ MALE _____
                MARRIED
                JOB SIMILAR TO CARPENTER OR BEAUTICIAN (CRAFTSMAN)
          _____ PT. "SOMETIMES" GETS NERVOUS OR UPSET _____
                PT. IDENTIFIED PROBLEM WITH BACK
                    SPINE
_____ PAIN, BURNING _____
                    PAIN WORSE ON EXCITEMENT
                    PAIN WORSE AFTER EXERCISE
          _____ MOST PAIN IN BACK _____
                PT. HAS HAD UNIDENTIFIED TYPE OF INFECTION IN LAST
                    SIX MONTHS
                INJURED WITHIN LAST YEAR _____
                PT. HAS HAD AN OPERATION ON:
                    STOMACH
          _____ DIZZY SPELLS IN LAST SIX MONTHS _____
                    SKIN SEEMS DRY
                PT. BRUISES EASILY
          _____ CHANGE IN SLEEPING HABITS _____
                PT. IDENTIFIES EITHER NUMBNESS, TINGLING OR ATAXIA
                PT. HAS FELT EITHER NERVOUS, DEPRESSED, OR
          _____    IRRITABLE LATELY. _____
                PT. HAS HAD PAIN IN THE HEAD OR HEADACHES IN THE
                    LAST SIX MONTHS.
          _____ PT. HAS PAIN OR TENDERNESS IN THE TOP OF THE HEAD. __
                    PAIN IS THROBBING
                    ASPIRIN OR HEADACHE TABLETS RELIEVE PAIN
          _____ PT. HAS A PROBLEM WITH HIS MOUTH, WITH BEING ___
                        THIRSTY, OR WITH HIS THROAT.
                PT. HAS A PROBLEM WITH HIS THROAT
          _____ PT. THROAT IS DRY OR SORE _____
                PT. OFTEN CHOKES OR GAGS
                PT. IDENTIFIED IRREGULAR HEART ACTION
          _____ PT. IDENTIFIED PROBLEM WITH APPETITE, DIGESTION OR __
                STOMACH
                PT. HAS NO CHANGE IN APPETITE
          _____ MILK OR FOOD RELIEVES PAIN _____
                FATTY FOOD CAUSES STOMACHACHE LASTING HOURS
                PT. BELCHES "A LOT"
          _____ PT. GETS "BLOWN UP" WITH GAS OR WIND _____
                PT. IDENTIFIED BURNING, CRAMPING, FULLNESS OR
                    PRESSURE IN STOMACH
          _____ NO REDNESS, STIFFNESS, SWELLING, OR PAIN IN JOINTS _____
                PT. IS NOT TIRED, WEAK, OR LIFELESS
                PT. HAS NOT FELT RESTLESS LATELY
          ___ PT. HAS NO UNUSUAL BLEEDING OR DISCHARGE _____
                PT. HAS NO PROBLEMS WITH NECK OR BACK
                NO NAUSEA OR VOMITING
          _____ PT. HAS NO WEIGHT CHANGE _____
                PT. HAS NOT HAD ANYTHING TO EAT OR DRINK IN PAST 3 HOURS
```

Figure 5.

identifies his symptoms and chief cause of complaint. The typewriter-like device has an associated audio-visual unit which reinforces the displayed text form of the question with a slide cartoon and with the recorded voice of the doctor. The patient interacts directly with the computer via the terminal for this test.

Figure 6 illustrates the report of the results of chemical laboratory tests made on a sample of blood drawn from the above patient. The blood is drawn in the clinic, transported to Columbia via courier and analyzed using an automated analyzer. The results are entered into the computer by a laboratory technician using a typewriter-like terminal. Similar printouts are obtained for hematologic results.

```
ATP REPORT 01/18/71 00:0C  0001724                        LAB REPORT

     AGE: 63
     SEX: MALE
     TEST              NORMAL RANGE         LAB RESULT

 —CHEMISTRY

     PATIENT IS FASTING
     CALCIUM            8.5 - 10.5                  10.3
     INORGANIC PHOSPHATE 2.5 - 4.5                   3.0
     GLUCOSE            65.0 - 110.0                95.0
     UREA NITROGEN      10 - 20                       12
     URIC ACID          2.5 - 8.6                    5.0
     CHOLESTEROL        150 - 300                    250
     TOTAL PROTEIN      6.0 - 8.0                   8.5 *
     ALBUMIN            3.5 - 5.0                    4.8
     TOTAL BILIRUBIN    .2 - 1.0                      .5
     ALKALINE PHOS.     30 - 85                       47
     LDH                80 - 200                     175
     SGOT               10 - 50                       27
```

Figure 6.

Electrocardiograms taken and recorded in the physician's office are transmitted to Columbia by telephone, where they are analyzed by the digital computer. The results are entered automatically into the computer file and are then available to the physician via a summary printout.

The results of a complete physician examination given by Dr. Bass are entered into the computer file by means of the terminal by a medical secretary. The results are printed out on three pages of which Figure 7 is illustrative.

```
O    ATP REPORT 01/18/71 10:30  0001724                    PHYS EX

                  ─── HEAD ───
O                    NORMAL

                  ─── HAIR COLOR ───
O                    GREY

                  ─── HAIR LOSS ───
O                    MILD

                  ─── SKIN ───
O                    LIGHT COMPLECTED
                     SMALL SCAR LT. TEMPLE AT HAIRLINE.

                  EYE MOVEMENT
O                     COORDINATED
                  ─── STEADY ───

                  CONJUNCTIVA
O                 ─── NORMAL ───

                  CORNEAS
O                    NORMAL

                  PUPILS
                  ─── ROUND, REGULAR & EQUAL ───
O                    NORMAL REACTION TO LIGHT
                     NORMAL REACTION TO ACCOMODATION

                  FUNDOSCOPY, RIGHT
O                    NORMAL
                  ─── MINUS LENS ───
O                    CLEAR MEDIA
                     NORMAL VISUAL RETINA
                  ─── NORMAL DISC ───

O

                  FUNDOSCOPY, LEFT
O                    NORMAL

                  EARS, EXTERNAL
O                    NORMAL

                  EAR CANAL, RIGHT
                     PATENT
                  ─── OTHER ───
O                    WAX PRESENT

                  ─── EAR CANAL, LEFT ───
O                    OBSTRUCTED, WAX

                  ─── EAR DRUMS ───
O                    NORMAL

                  AIR CONDUCTION
O                    ABNORMAL RIGHT
                  ─── ABNORMAL LEFT ───

O
```

Figure 7.

The "vital signs" are taken and recorded by the nurse and entered into the fil via the terminal. The blood pressure values are obtained from an automated blood pressure machine equipped with a digital read-out for ease of operation. Height, weight, temperature, pulse rate, respiration rate and blood pressure are printed out.

Another printout shows the results of a hearing test taken by an automatic recording audiometer. This device is a discrete frequency audiometer which automatically displays the patient's pure tone air

```
ATP REPORT 03/10/71 16:29  0001724                              COMMENTS
THIS 63 YEAR OLD MALE WAS REFERRED FOR EVALUATION ON 2/15/71 BY
DR. BILLY BASS, SALEM, MISSOURI.  THE ADMITTING PROBLEM WAS THAT OF
A RIGHT PULMONARY INFILTRATE.  THE PATIENT GAVE A HISTORY OF
PNEUMONIA IN 1963 WITH RECURRING EPISODES IN 1970 AND 1971.  THE 1971
EPISODE OCCURRED IN JANUARY AND WITH THAT EPISODE, FOR THE FIRST TIME,
THE PATIENT EXPERIENCED HEMOPTYSIS, WHICH CONTINUED UNTIL ONE WEEK
PRIOR TO ADMISSION.  EXCEPT FOR THE RECENT DEVELOPMENT OF DYSPNEA ON
EXERTION, THE PATIENT HAD NO SYSTEMIC SYMPTOMS.  PREOPERATIVE EVALUA-
TION WAS WITHIN NORMAL LIMITS EXCEPT FOR A BRONCHOGRAM ON 2/17/71
WHICH DEMONSTRATED AMPUTATION OF THE ANTERIOR BASILAR SEGMENTAL
BRONCHUS ON THE RIGHT WITH SOME NARROWING AND IRREGULARITY OF THE
WALL OF THE MEDIAL BASILAR SEGMENTAL BRONCHUS, THESE FINDINGS MOST
LIKELY DUE TO CARCINOMA OF THE ANTERIOR BASILAR SEGMENT WITH SECONDARY
INFLAMMATORY REACTION INVOLVING ADJACENT STRUCTURES.  BRONCHIAL BIOPSY
CARRIED OUT ON 2/18/71 WAS REPORTED AS DEMONSTRATING SQUAMOUS CELL
CARCINOMA, BRONCHOGENIC, WELL DIFFERENTIATED, IN THE RIGHT LOWER LOBE
BRONCHUS.  PREOPERATIVE ELECTROCARDIOGRAM DEMONSTRATED  NODAL PREMATURE
BEATS, BUT WAS OTHERWISE WITHIN NORMAL LIMITS AND CARDIOLOGY CLEARANCE
FOR RESECTION WAS GRANTED.  PREOPERATIVE PULMONARY FUNCTION STUDIES
DEMONSTRATED A MAXIMUM BREATHING CAPACITY OF 69 LITERS PER MINUTE AS
OPPOSED TO A NORMAL OF 98, AND A ONE SECOND TIMED VITAL CAPACITY OF
62% AS OPPOSED TO 81%.  DESPITE THIS, HE HAD GOOD EXERCISE TOLERANCE
IN A SIMPLE STAIR CLIMBING TEST SUGGESTING THAT HE WAS A BORDERLINE
CANDIDATE FOR PNEUMONECTOMY BUT PROBABLY WOULD TOLERATE LOBECTOMY OR
BILOBECTOMY SATISFACTORILY.  ON 2/25/71, A RIGHT LOWER LOBECTOMY WAS
CARRIED OUT.  IT WAS NOT POSSIBLE TO DETERMINE PRIOR TO BEGINNING
THE LOBECTOMY THAT THE TUMOR WAS UNRESECTABLE BECAUSE OF PERIBRONCHIAL
EXTENSION OF THE TUMOR AND BY THE TIME THAT THIS HAD BEEN DETERMINED
WITH CERTAINTY, LOBECTOMY WAS NECESSARY.  THE IMMEDIATE POSTOPERATIVE
COURSE WAS COMPLICATED BY MASSIVE BLEEDING INTO THE RIGHT CHEST FROM
THE INFERIOR PULMONARY VEIN REQUIRING EARLY SECONDARY THORACOTOMY FOR
CONTROL OF BLEEDING.  THE PATIENT TOLERATED BOTH SURGICAL PROCEDURES
SATISFACTORILY, AND THE PATIENT WAS DISCHARGED HOME ON 3/5/71 WITH
AN APPOINTMENT TO RADIATION THERAPY.  HE WAS SEEN IN RADIATION THERAPY
ON MARCH 8, 1971, AT WHICH TIME IT WAS RECOMMENDED THAT POSTOPERATIVE
SUPPLEMENTARY RADIATION THERAPY WAS JUSTIFIED FOR RESIDUAL TUMOR AROUND
THE PULMONARY ARTERY, VEINS, AND NEXT TO THE RIGHT ATRIUM SINCE THERE
WAS NO EVIDENCE OF DISTANT METASTASIS, CLINICALLY OR RADIOGRAPHICALLY.

DIAGNOSIS:   SQUAMOUS CELL CARCINOMA, RIGHT LOWER LOBE, BROCHOGENIC
             CHRONIC RIGHT LOWER LOBE ATALECTASIS

OPERATIONS:  BRONCHOSCOPY AND RIGHT LOWER LOBE BIOPSY, 2/18/71
             RIGHT LOWER LOBECTOMY, 2/25/71
             EMERGENCY SECONDARY THORACOTOMY FOR BLEEDING, 2/25/71

             CARL H. ALMOND, M.D. CHIEF, SECTION OF THORACIC AND
                                  CARDIOVASCULAR SURGERY
```

Figure 8.

conduction thresholds in a form giving hearing loss at each of six different frequencies. The nurse records these values and enters them into the computer file via the terminal.

The results of a vision test which measures visual acuity, color perception and lateral and vertical phoria are similarly administered by the nurse; the data entered into the computer file can be printed out on request.

Similar procedures are used in obtaining the report of the x-ray examination as entered by the consulting radiologist. The x-ray is taken in the clinic and transported to Columbia by a courier service.

Comments entered by the physician after reviewing all of the information contained in the other sections of the summary report are printed out.

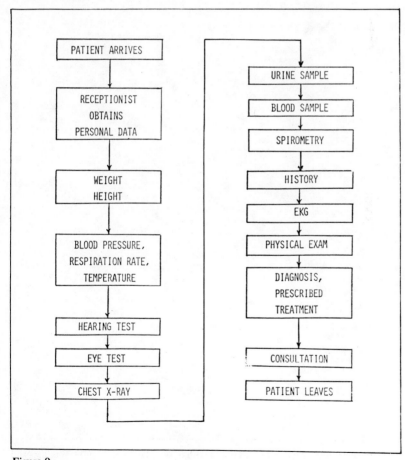

Figure 9.

Figure 8 shows a summary of tests, findings and treatments administered to this patient upon admission to the University of Missouri Medical
Center in Columbia. He has now returned to his home in Salem and is
recovering satisfactorily.

Figure 9 is a flow diagram of the typical order in which the patient
takes the battery of tests. All patients do not necessarily take all of the
tests.

The major goals of the present testing program are to modify the
system to be more useful to the physician; to redesign the system to be
more cost effective; and to evaluate the potential use of the system in
metropolitan areas, solo practices, group practices and clinics.

This work was supported by Public Health Service Grant RM00009. Findings and
conclusions do not necessarily represent the views of the U. S. Public Health Service.

The Automated AFEES Project

Rudolf G. Bickel

The Automated Armed Forces Examining and Entrance Stations (AFEES) project is a computer-based physical examination and processing system for the Armed Forces. Development and operational testing of the 100-man-per-day pilot system will occur during the next three to four years. Decisions will then be made as to further implementation of this concept in AFEES and for other routine and periodic physical examinations.

This Department of Defense-directed project resulted in part from needs and requirements identified by a Tri-Service Working Group for the Modernization of Routine Physical Examinations (MORPE). These requirements included an increase in the accuracy, validity and quality of the examination; the ability to complete record forms automatically; an improvement in the storage and retrieval of records; the provision of needed statistical data; and possession of capability for growth, modification and expansion.

These general criteria were formulated for all routine physicals in the DOD and have served as key guidelines during this specific development of the AFEES. Other objectives were added to the Statement of Work to meet specific user needs and specific DOD requirements. These additional requirements are (1) the satisfaction of all examination and processing requirements, (2) the ability to accommodate 100 examinees in six hours, (3) the flexibility to accommodate female applicants, (4) the accomplishment of scheduling and administrative procedures, (5) the provision of positive examinee identification, and (6) the ability to provide a printed history and physical examination available for signature the same day the examination occurred.

Additional AFEES Requirements

This project was known as AMES (Automated Medical Examination System) during the study phase, which perhaps implied that only

Rudolf G. Bickel, Major, USAF, MC, *Chief, Medical Systems Development Branch, Medical Systems Division, United States Air Force School of Aerospace Medicine, Brooks Air Force Base, Tex.*

medically related functions were involved. Since the entire processing function is, in fact, included in this project, the name has been changed to Automated AFEES to more clearly reflect this fact.

The USAF School of Aerospace Medicine (USAFSAM), along with its systems analysis consultants from Hq Electronic Systems Division at Hanscom Field, Massachusetts, prepared an overall development plan. This plan was approved and the USAFSAM subsequently became the lead organization for Phase 1 of this development.

The development plan involves three phases. Phase 1 was a definition of the pilot system and involved obtaining the mission analysis, conducting state-of-the-art surveys, identifying promising methods for possible research and development, developing a preliminary systems plan and possible options, and delivering a detailed final systems plan. Phase 2 is the development, fabrication and installation of the pilot system. Finally, Phase 3 will be a one-year operational test and evaluation of the system.

The Statement of Work required that the Phase 1 study contractor, Philco-Ford Western Development Laboratories, first accomplish a complete mission analysis of several AFEES, so as to fully appreciate all operational needs and requirements. Next, the contractor was asked to study the state of the art for all equipment and procedures – medical, administrative and ancillary – that could possibly accomplish necessary improvements identified either by the Statement of Work or in the AFEES Mission Analysis. At this time, the contractor also recommended areas in which specific additional studies or developments could lead to techniques or methods that would be potentially useful to the AFEES. Comments from the DOD agencies involved were incorporated in the additional guidance to the contractor. We received the final volume of the completed system plan in November 1970. These reports will serve as a firm foundation for decisions concerning exact system details and for developing and installing the prototype system.

Final approval to proceed for Phases 2 and 3 has been given by the DOD and the Air Force. During Phase 2, Electronic Systems Division will have prime responsibility for the overall development, with the Medical Systems Division providing support on all medically related elements. Phase 3 will represent a one-year operational test under full load by the using organization, The US Army Recruiting Command (USAREC).

It should be pointed out that the need for the study phase was questioned at regular intervals, particularly by those who felt that they had "off the shelf" multiphasic health screening (MPHS) systems fully capable of meeting our needs. However, while AFEES processing has a few features common to the HEW-sponsored and commercial demonstration MPHS system, it differs in many others. The AFEES examination is accomplished on 19-year-olds to determine physical fitness for military service. MPHS systems typically screen 40-, 50-, and 60-year-olds to detect diseases which are usually far less common in young men; thus, even the medical aspects differ considerably. In AFEES, the unpredictable daily workload may more than double; yet the work, including a final physician evaluation, must still be completed the same day. The heavy and complex AFEES administrative burden is of a far different nature than at civilian clinics; in fact, it represents the major portion of the AFEES workload at present. Many aspects, such as learning aptitudes testing, e.g., the Armed Forces Qualification Test (AFQT), are also unique to AFEES.

Although certain components of existing systems will doubtless be suitable for AFEES needs, it should be clear that no "off the shelf" system has been designed to fill these specialized demands. And, because this is a new kind of system, we cannot at this time fully predict every detail of the actual pilot system.

However, we have a firm basis upon which to make the necessary decisions during development. The contractor's studies were honest and thorough and will serve as a solid point of departure. In-house studies during the study phase independently validated many contractor conclusions. These have continued and have more completely defined needed tasks in many critical areas.

A third study was performed in-house following a request from DOD for detailed costs and specific causes of discharges for conditions existing prior to service (EPTS). As a result of this highly detailed study, we now know areas of the medical processing that must receive additional emphasis and what the precise nature of the emphasis must be.

The contractor's design concept shows what his system proposes and what kinds of things it contains (Fig. 1). This system configuration was selected after considering some 28 different design concepts, ranging from the present manual system to the most sophisticated automation now possible. After reviewing various concepts and possible means to accomplish each required task within the system, this proved to be the most cost-effective design having all desired characteristics.

The contractor's design concept includes real time data entry and status control. Data are inserted in varying ways: teletypewriter terminals for administrative information, a mark sense reader for history and AFQT scoring, cathode ray tube terminals for physicians' data. Stations measuring functions such as height, weight, visual acuity and the like enter observations directly into the computer whenever feasible, although some stations may have small manual entry terminals. A special examinee's ID badge is used when data are entered to assure correct assignment. Microfilm records contain non-machine-codable information, such as

AMES SYSTEM PLAN

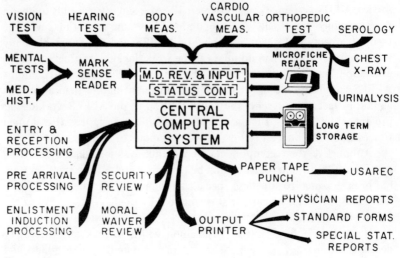

Figure 1.

referring physician letters, and it also provides a permanent record of all machine-printed forms and signed documents relating to an individual.

Data output includes automated printing of most forms, including administrative forms now typed by hand, the SF 88 and the 89 or 93, as well as summaries and reports. Magnetic tapes retain information for later statistical analysis.

What will this system do for the physician and for the accuracy, reliability, and validity of the examination recorded? First, the system will include *improved examination techniques* for a number of measurements – such as blood pressure, height and weight.

Second, it will provide *improved medical information transmittal* in the areas of legibility (need I say more?), accuracy (using direct entry whenever feasible and providing internal calibration routines and checks), and validity.

Third, it will give a more functional presentation of information to the physician, who must now scan each handwritten entry to detect the few abnormal findings buried among the mass of normal data. This can be done by flagging items suggesting disease or indicating additional tests of consultation; flagging out-of-limits results for physical standards of the class of examination being performed; flagging incomplete results, to keep the examinations from being inadvertently released as completed; and flagging inconsistent results (e.g., inconsistent answers to history questions, history-physical examination inconsistencies).

Fourth, it will provide a more functional entry of information by physicians. Based on systems now in use at civilian medical centers, an easy-to-use branching display and data entry system will be developed and modified for AFEES needs. This will permit the physician to describe completely, consistently and legibly most history and examination findings, both normal and abnormal. Narrative descriptions of rare findings or of any additional details would, of course, continue. This capability will permit valid comparisons with future examinations, since one man's "3+" will not then have to be compared with another's "four finger breadths," or another's "markedly." And, for the first time, it will permit a valid analysis of medical characteristics of the populations seen in AFEES. Since the resulting physical examination report will be codable by the computer, it can easily be used to study characteristics of examinees. Currently, the only consistent examination terminology in the SF 88 is "normal" and "abnormal," and the rest, in "free text," is not amenable to such studies.

Fifth, the system will provide *assistance with pertinent regulations and standards,* with displays of suggested examination protocols or decision criteria immediately available on request. This will provide consistency throughout the various AFEES and will in particular ease the problems of newly assigned physicians.

Sixth, the system will provide *quality control* because of its capability to audit results.

Finally, perhaps the most important goal of this system is that it can *produce a valid, usable data base* for later medical evaluation and care of the examinee. It would be of great value to both the individual and his physician if the routine physical examination provided clinically useful baseline information. Few clinicians trust the information presently recorded during routine physical examinations and fewer use it for patient care. If the content and reliability of these examinations would permit them to be integrated into an ongoing medical data base for later clinical use, overall health care would be significantly enhanced.

Many administrative functions will be improved. In fact, the greatest AFEES manpower savings will result from improvements in this area. Since most of these benefits, such as automatic form completion with avoidance of transcription errors, are relatively obvious, I shall not discuss them in detail.

The Automated AFEES pilot system must serve a dual role: as a prototype for future systems of its kind, and as a test bed to validate new concepts, methods and devices. Thus, the basic system design must be kept flexible so that it can grow gracefully as needed. Independent estimates of total costs per year of this pilot system design, made by the contractor and by the Air Force, show that the cost per examinee of the contractor's recommended design for the pilot Automated AFEES will be very close to that of the present manual system, despite the additional flexibility and complexity needed for a test and development system. Costs for follow-on systems will, of course, depend on their design and other factors not yet firmly established.

Let me speak for a moment of the broad goals of this development. The immediate goal is clearly better detection of significant disease conditions and better implementation and definition of physical standards, along with a more effective use of medical manpower. A secondary gain, that of a decreased number of unfit individuals entering the service, may result in considerable cost savings due to the decreased number of EPTS discharges. Cost savings in AFEES operations may also occur but cannot yet be confirmed.

Long-term goals and implications must include providing better routine examinations of all kinds to all those eligible for military medical care, with a resulting improvement in the quality of health care provided. For these goals to be achieved, changes in the practice of medicine and in many aspects of medical records must be anticipated. The data base resulting from routine examinations must be so structured that it becomes a useful, reliable, vital part of the medical record. Only then will it form a firm foundation for understanding the patient's problems and for his comprehensive and episodic care requirements.

The views expressed herein are those of the author and do not necessarily reflect the views of the U.S. Air Force or the Department of Defense.

AMHTS and the VA Admission Procedure

Richard E. Gordon, Charles Holzer, Leslie Bielen, Anne Watts and Katherine L. Gordon

In the Gainesville VA Hospital, the admission decision is a crucial one. Eligible veterans receive in-patient care if needed, but are expected to obtain out-patient services mostly from sources other than the VA since the latter has limited out-patient facilities. Thus, the admitting physician has an important responsibility in deciding whether or not the patient's condition requires and will benefit from in-patient hospital services.

Many veterans receive, or hope to receive, pensions from the Government for their disabilities. This compensation, which in effect rewards illness, naturally tends to evoke symptoms which usually date back to the period in which the veteran was in service. This study will also explore the potential usefulness of AMHTS in helping the admission physician separate the truly sick from the merely symptomatic.

Method

Veterans were tested by AMHTS while they were undergoing the admission process at the Gainesville VA Hospital. Testing was voluntary and 212 patients of the 795 contacted agreed to be screened. Of these, 123 were subsequently admitted to the hospital (Adm Group), and 83 were not admitted to the hospital (Non-Adm Group). Follow-up was not available on six patients. Patients, when they agreed to be tested, did not know whether they were going to be admitted. Admitting physicians did not receive any information about the patients' test results until after the admission procedure had been completed and the patients were either sent home or admitted to the ward.

In order not to fail to provide care to someone who truly needed it, the AMHTS printout on all patients was subsequently delivered to the chief admitting physician. On the basis of findings on these printouts, three patients of the Non-Adm Group who previously had been refused

Richard E. Gordon, M.D., Ph.D., Charles Holzer, B.A., Leslie Bielen, M.Ed., Anne Watts, D.A.S.S. *and* Katherine L. Gordon, *Department of Psychiatry, University of Florida College of Medicine, Gainesville, Fla.*

116   R. E. GORDON ET AL.

admission were called back and admitted for hospital care. Two of these patients had abnormalities on their chest x-ray and another had electrocardiogram abnormalities. In this study they remain part of the Non-Adm Group.

In the admitting office, the decision whether to admit has been made after consultation with physicians from the specialty services involved. We have divided these patients, therefore, into three primary groups — medicine and the medical specialties, surgery and its specialties, and psychiatry. There were 42 admissions to the medical services and 35 non-admissions; 60 surgical admissions and 33 non-admissions; 21 psychiatric admissions and 15 non-admissions. Many patients received consultations from other services than the primary one responsible for admission. In every case we kept patients in their primary category — even when admission was to another group.

The AMHTS battery consists of the tests and procedures shown in Table 1, all of which are reported in summary form on the computer printout.

Comparisons were made between admitted and non-admitted patients by means of X^2 and t-tests. As can be seen in Table 1 by inspection of the number of items and the value of the means, the questionnaire scores approximate the Poisson distribution. The square roots of the scores should approximate the normal distribution. In calculating differences by means of t-tests between admitted and non-admitted VA patients, and correlations between items, we have therefore utilized the square root of each score.

Except for psychiatric patients, the ages of admitted and non-admitted patients were similar. Nine of 21 psychiatric admissions (43%) were in their twenties or younger as compared to 11 of the 102 (11%) admitted on the other services. As for the numbers of black and white patients admitted to each service, there were no racial differences between admitted and non-admitted patients.

The sample of patients screened is likely to be biased. With the decision to take part in AMHTS a voluntary one for patients recruited in the Admitting Area, patients who were especially anxious and concerned with physical symptoms and medical history were more likely to cooperate.

Nevertheless, the cross tabulation by race, age, disposition and service, even when the differences do not reach significant levels statistically, are useful to describe the nature of the patient population and to point the direction for future studies. Although the values are not necessarily an indication of pathology, they do show differences between admitted and non-admitted patients and between those in the different services.

TABLE 1. Instrumental Tests

On Line	Chemistry	Hematology
Systolic BP	BUN	WBC
Diastolic BP	Creatinine	RBC
Spirometry (raw) FEV 0.5	Bilirubin	Hemoglobin
Spirometry (raw) FEV 1.0	Proteins	Hematocrit
Spirometry (raw) FVC	Cholesterol	MCV
Tonometry, left eye	Uric Acid	MCHC
Tonometry, right eye	Glucose	MCH
EKG (normal, abnormal)		
	Chest x-ray	

Questionnaire Systems

Sum	Number of Items	Mean
Family history	18	2.5
Infectious disease	14	3.3
Illnesses	24	2.2
Operations	14	1.1
Allergies	8	0.3
Emotional	16	5.5
General	12	2.9
Male problems	4	0.4
Gastrointestinal	24	3.1
Headaches	12	2.1
Respiratory	12	2.6
Cardiology	19	4.2
Genito-urinary	12	1.2
Ear-nose-throat	13	2.5
Neurological	13	2.9
Musculoskeletal	10	2.4
Ophthalmology	8	1.5
	233	40.7
Life Crisis Score		132.3

In order to measure the extent of overreporting of symptoms by veterans, a group of VA patients was compared to a comparable group of patients at the Shands Teaching Hospital. AMHTS results of 60 Shands Hospital patients who were screened prior to admission for eye surgery were analyzed and compared to a similar group of 15 veterans. Patients in both groups were matched by age and compared on the basis of their chemical and physiological findings to determine how well they were matched as to actual physical health. Then their responses to the history questionnaire were compared by numbers of symptoms per system. It was hypothesized that veterans would present significantly greater numbers of complaints per system and totally than would non-veteran hospital patients.

Results

Admitted VA patients differed from those who were refused admission on a number of AMHTS tests. In general, admitted patients reported more symptoms on the AMHTS history questionnaire than non-admitted (Table 2). Differences were particularly significant for patients admitted to the medical services, with special reference to symptoms associated with neurological, musculoskeletal, respiratory and ENT systems; those of a general nature; and those associated with past illnesses. Surgical patients, on the other hand, with larger numbers of respiratory and musculoskeletal symptoms were not likely to be admitted. Psychiatric patients reporting allergies were not admitted (Table 3).

With respect to findings from the physiological and chemical tests and examinations, it appeared that, except in the case of diastolic blood pressure where patients with higher blood pressure tended not to be admitted, there were few significant differences between the entire group of admitted patients and those not admitted. However, when test results were studied for each of the three major services, a number of differences

TABLE 2. Questionnaire Items

	Admitted Mean (N = 123)	Non-Admitted Mean (N = 83)
Family history	2.6*	2.3
Infectious diseases	3.3	3.4
Illnesses	2.4*	2.0
Operations	1.1	1.1
Allergies	0.3	0.3
Male problems	0.5*	0.3
Gastrointestinal	3.5*	2.7
Headaches	2.4*	1.9
Respiratory	2.6	2.7
Cardiovascular	4.2	4.4
Ear-nose-throat	2.4	2.8
Genito-urinary	1.4*	1.0
Neurological	3.0*	2.9
Musculoskeletal	2.4	2.4
Ophthalmology	1.6*	1.5
Emotional	5.8*	5.2
General symptoms	3.1*	2.6
Total Sum	42.6*	39.5
Rahe & Homes	129.3	136.7

*With ten systems and the total symptom score, admitted patients had higher mean scores than non-admitted patients; three mean scores were the same, and in four instances mean symptom scores of admitted patients were less than those of non-admitted.

TABLE 3. Comparisons by Service of Questionnaire Responses of Adm and Non-Adm VA Patients Where Differences Occurred

		Admitted Mean Sq Rt	S.D.	Non-Admitted Mean Sq Rt	S.D.	t	
Illnesses	All	1.41	0.66	1.20	0.75	2.17	0.05
	Med	1.48	0.73	1.08	0.80	2.51	near 0.01
	Surg	1.32	0.64	1.24	0.72		
	Psy	1.52	0.54	1.65	0.41		
Allergy	All	0.25	0.47	0.26	0.47		
	Med	0.17	0.41	0.20	0.42		
	Surg	0.31	0.51	0.22	0.45		
	Psy	0.26	0.49	0.72	0.64	1.97	0.05
Ear, Nose, Throat	All	2.23	0.89	2.15	0.77		
	Med	2.34	0.80	2.00	0.83	1.92	near 0.05
	Surg	2.03	0.88	2.11	0.58		
	Psy	2.65	0.99	3.03	0.63		
General	All	1.66	0.64	1.52	0.53		
	Med	1.77	0.58	1.55	0.57	1.69	0.10
	Surg	1.50	0.68	1.44	0.50		
	Psy	1.91	0.50	1.73	0.40		
Neurological	All	1.31	1.16	1.31	1.10		
	Med	1.51	1.22	1.03	1.03	1.98	0.05
	Surg	1.16	1.05	1.54	1.13	1.63	0.10
	Psy	1.33	1.32	1.80	1.13		
Musculo-skeletal	All	1.13	1.04	1.26	0.93		
	Med	1.23	1.03	1.08	0.96		
	Surg	1.06	1.04	1.61	0.80	2.61	0.01
	Psy	1.11	1.09	0.82	0.90		
Respiratory	All	1.28	1.00	1.29	1.02		
	Med	1.57	0.93	1.21	1.08	1.68	0.10
	Surg	1.00	1.02	1.34	0.96	1.62	0.10
	Psy	1.50	0.90	1.46	1.06		

appeared between admitted and refused patients. In most cases, patients who were not admitted were more likely to have abnormal findings. This was the case among psychiatric patients with respect to systolic blood pressure readings, hemoglobin, hematocrit, uric acid and mean corpuscular hemoglobin concentration. Admitted surgical patients also had poor spirometry values (Table 4).

A number of tests were also analyzed for abnormal and normal values by means of X^2:

1. For blood proteins, ten of 108 admitted patients (9%) had levels above 8.2 grams % in comparison to 17 of 81 (21%) who were not admitted. ($X^2 = 5.4$ p < 0.05)
2. On the Rahe and Holmes test, medical patients with higher Life Crisis scores were more likely to be admitted. Among those

TABLE 4. Comparisons by Service of Physiological and Chemical Test Findings of Adm and Non-Adm VA Patients Where Differences Occurred

		Admitted		Non-Admitted			
		Mean	S.D.	Mean	S.D.	t	p
Systolic BP	All	129.30	37.39	136.71	32.11		
	Med	134.20	34.76	140.12	24.19		
	Surg	128.73	40.24	140.12	40.64		
	Psy	118.06	32.91	140.50	29.73	1.65	0.10
Diastolic	All	70.46	23.50	78.45	23.92	2.35	0.05
BP	Med	76.76	20.29	82.17	26.24		
	Surg	66.92	24.97	73.30	22.15		
	Psy	65.88	23.84	80.13	14.68		
Spirometry	All	199.62	74.07	190.53	81.10		
FEV 0.5	Med	176.73	70.25	183.91	86.43		
	Surg	212.20	76.10	183.81	77.32	1.69	0.10
	Psy	210.72	66.64	221.50	74.65		
Spirometry	All	298.49	101.55	302.39	108.68		
FEV 1.0	Med	262.93	104.13	288.15	112.83		
	Surg	319.30	97.10	289.41	102.12		
	Psy	310.58	93.17	365.64	97.07	1.65	0.10
Creatinine	All	1.177	0.238	1.20	0.266		
	Med	1.085	0.193	1.313	0.340	2.25	0.05
	Surg	1.184	0.229	1.167	0.231		
	Psy	1.30	0.266	1.10	0.187		
Proteins	All	7.566	0.576	7.781	0.534	2.62	0.01
	Med	7.658	0.74	7.83	0.598		
	Surg	7.511	0.481	7.721	0.537		
	Psy	7.572	0.521	7.807	0.354		
Uric Acid	All	5.675	1.528	5.602	1.502		
	Med	5.381	1.712	5.571	1.633		
	Surg	5.822	1.496	5.858	1.538		
	Psy	5.790	1.22	5.113	0.960	1.78	0.10
Glucose	All	151.94	66.97	176.00	65.59	2.50	near 0.01
	Med	144.10	70.04	174.03	57.43		
	Surg	159.93	61.82	184.29	66.85		
	Psy	144.85	75.30	163.47	81.83		
Hemoglobin	All	15.099	1.529	15.273	1.441		
	Med	15.143	1.443	15.026	1.586		
	Surg	15.082	1.626	15.124	1.369		
	Psy	15.061	1.468	16.160	0.873	2.55	near 0.01
Hematocrit	All	45.34	4.37	45.70	3.79		
	Med	45.63	4.21	45.09	4.29		
	Surg	45.04	4.56	45.30	3.48		
	Psy	45.68	4.30	47.93	2.31	1.83	0.10
MCHC	All	33.71	1.12	33.76	1.12		
	Med	33.59	1.21	33.68	0.98		
	Surg	33.95	1.06	33.70	1.24		
	Psy	33.17	0.92	34.07	1.16	2.48	0.05
Specific	All	1016.88	6.68	1018.00	5.89		
Gravity	Med	1016.20	7.67	1019.12	5.15	1.88	0.10
	Surg	1018.19	5.78	1017.03	5.56		
	Psy	1014.55	6.49	1017.50	8.14		

medical patients who were admitted to the medical services, 15 of
37 (40.5%) had scores higher than 249 in comparison to six out of
31 (19%) who were not admitted. $(X^2 = 6$ p $< 0.05)$

3. With x-ray, four out of five (80%) psychiatric patients who were
admitted had abnormal chest films in comparison to one of
eight (12.5%) of the non-admitted psychiatric patients.
$(X^2 = 4.7$ p $< 0.05)$

4. Patients with blood cholesterol levels higher than 231 were
significantly less likely to be admitted to the surgery service. Only
20 of the 57 (35%) admitted patients had blood levels higher than
230 in comparison to 19 of 33 (58%) of those not admitted.
$(X^2 = 4.3$ p $< 0.05)$

5. Patients with glucose levels above 200 were more likely not to be
admitted on any of the services. Of these, 20 out of 111 (28%)
were admitted and 31 of 80 (39%) were not admitted.
$(X^2 = 6.8$ p $< 0.01)$

Age tended to be a factor in patient admissions, especially with older
patients. In general, elderly patients (those past 60 years of age) who were
not admitted tended to have a significant number of higher system scores
on their symptom questionnaires and abnormal test findings than did the
admitted elderly. The reverse was true of middle aged patients (aged 30 to
59). No differences were seen with young patients (29 or less in age)
(Table 5).

As shown in Table 6, veteran patients presented more than twice as
many symptoms as did non-veteran eye patients on the AMHTS
questionnaire. This was a fact in the case of every system except allergy.
On the other hand, except for systolic blood pressure, non-veteran eye
patients of the same age at the Shands Teaching Hospital had more
abnormal findings on the physiological and chemical tests (Table 7),
suggesting that as a group they actually were physically sicker.

Discussion

The patient's history and symptoms apparently were related to the
physician's admission decision. Thus, AMHTS testing might help him by
saving time. It also appears that if certain AMHTS test data were available,
the physicians might be assisted in coming to a better decision. As
mentioned earlier, several Non-Adm subjects were called back for
subsequent admission because of EKG and Chest x-ray abnormalities
found on the AMHTS workup.

It would seem that the decision as to which service works up a patient
has a bearing on the likelihood of his admission. It is conceivable that the
AMHTS printout would assist the admitting physician in assigning patients

122   R. E. GORDON ET AL.

TABLE 5. Questionnaire and Test Scores Which Discriminated Between Adm and Non-Adm VA Patients of Different Ages

Young Patients (29 years or less)
None

Middle Aged Patients (30-59)
    Higher Symptom Scores or Abnormal Test Results

Admitted	Non-Admitted
Illnesses**	None
Musculoskeletal***	
Ophthalmology**	
General*	
Tonometry*	

Elderly Patients (60 and older)
    Higher Symptom Scores or Abnormal Test Results

Admitted	Non-Admitted
General*	Blood glucose***
	Infectious disease*
	Cardiovascular**
	Ear-nose-throat*

Significant Level
   * 0.10
  ** 0.05
*** 0.01

TABLE 6. Comparisons by System of Questionnaire Responses of VA Versus Shands Teaching Hospital Eye Patients

	Shands Hospital $N = 17$ Mean	VA Hospital $N = 15$ Mean
Family history	1.8	2.33
Infectious diseases	2.6	3.27
Past illnesses	1.5	3.27
Operations	0.5	0.93
Allergies	0.4	0.27
Respiratory symptoms	1.5	2.33
Cardiovascular symptoms	1.4	4.4
GI complaints	0.5	2.533
G.U. symptoms	0.1	1.93
Neurological symptoms	0.4	2.47
Musculoskeletal symptoms	0.2	2.13
Ophthalmology	3.5	4.73
ENT symptoms	0.8	3.07
Headaches	0.8	3.20
Emotional complaints	2.5	5.0
General symptoms	1.8	2.93
Sexual problems	0.10	0.60
	20.4	44.7

TABLE 7. Comparisons by System of Physiological and Chemical
Test Findings of VA and Shands Hospital Eye Patients

	Shands Hospital N = 17 Overall Means	VA Hospital N = 15 Overall Means
Systolic BP	129.31	146.5*
Diastolic BP	78.94*	72.27
Spirometry		
0.5	1.64	1.68
1.0	2.50*	2.77
3.0	3.67*	4.05
Tonometry		
Right Eye	23.82*	16.40
Left Eye	23.47*	20.27
BUN	15.27	15.2
Creatinine	1.27	1.08
Bilirubin	0.99	1.03
Protein	7.10	7.60
Cholesterol	242.93*	228.33
Uric Acid	5.71	6.38
WBC	7.18	6.95
RBC	4.99	4.61
Hemoglobin	15.23	14.70
Hematocrit	45.88	44.33
MCV	92.63	92.00
MCH	30.75	31.87
MCHC	33.06	33.87

*More abnormal

to a service for workup, consultation, etc. In this way a broad range of medical information would be immediately available to the admitting physician. An awareness of the findings of the instrument tests could provide more information for the admission decision.

A comparison of AMHTS findings with veteran and non-veteran patients for eye surgery would indicate that the testing procedure might assist the admitting physician to some extent in assessing the significance of veteran patients' complaints. An AMHTS printout containing great numbers of symptoms referable to almost every system, but with few physiological and chemical abnormalities, would probably be revealing to the doctor who must assess the seriousness of a veteran's or other compensation patient's complaints.

We expect that the laboratory and other instrumental data may be of additional use in the initial workup of the patient on the ward along with the automated history part of the testing examination. This phase of the study has now begun and a report will be forthcoming.

The VA Hospital system, as Donald Johnson, Administrator of Veterans Affairs, points out, is America's largest hospital system under single management, containing 165 hospitals and 202 out-patient clinics, in addition to other facilities. Already, nearly half of the population is entitled or potentially entitled to VA benefits and services, either as veterans or as dependents or survivors of war veterans.

In this era when the public is increasingly expecting quality health care for everyone, Johnson recommends that the VA system serve as a "model for other systems that may be developed." He proposes that VA medicine can provide a "kind of health care laboratory in which new concepts for expanded preventive and ambulatory care can be perfected and then applied nationwide to relieve and ultimately reverse the present reliance upon in-hospital facilities." He suggests that VA medicine helps to develop methods that reverse or at least limit health care costs through efficient use of facilities and personnel. Perhaps AMHTS may eventually provide an example of one of the to-be-hoped-for new methods.

Acknowledgments

We appreciate the assistance of the following persons at the University of Florida and the Gainesville VA Hospital: Dr. Mario Ariet, Dr. Ewen Clark, Dr. H. G. Greenier, Dr. John Thornby, Dr. Ed. Cohen, Dr. George Warheit, Dr. Carolyn Hursch and Miss Anna Beiser.

This study was supported in part by Regional Medical Program Grant #PHS-RM-0024-92C and VA Grant #01/3210.1/69.01.

Bibliography

Bates, Barbara: Physicians use and opinions of screening tests in ambulatory practice. *JAMA*, 214:2173-2180, 1970.

Gordon, P. C.: Screening for disease in hospital and clinic populations. *Canad. J. Public Health*, 57:249-259, 1966.

Hilleboe, H. E. and Schaeffer, M.: Evaluation in community health: Relating results to goals. *Bull. N. Y. Acad. Med.*, 44:140-158, 1968.

Howe, H. F.: Medical problems in multiphasic screening. Paper presented at Engineering Foundation Conference on Multiphasic Screening, Deerfield, Mass., Aug. 18-22, 1969.

Johnson, D. E.: Remarks at the 50th New England Hospital Assembly, Boston, Mass., March 30, 1971.

Thorner, R. M.: Acceptance of multiphasic screening and the doctor-patient relationship. Paper presented at the Engineering Foundation Conference on Multiphasic Health Screening, Deerfield, Mass., Aug. 18-22, 1969.

Thorner, R. M.: Whither multiphasic screening. *New Eng. J. Med.*, 280:1037-1042, 1969.

Westlake, R. E.: Acceptance by and impact of screening on health professionals. *Bull. N. Y. Acad. Med.*, 45:1376-1383, 1969.

Williamson, J. W., Alexander, M. and Miller, G. E.: Continuing education and patient care research: Physician response to screening test results. *JAMA*, 201:938-942, 1967.

The Role of AMHT in Health Care Systems

James L. Craig

Introduction

Automated multiphasic health testing (AMHT) is a broad general term that has several definitions — depending on who and how someone is using automated systems for screening purposes. It has stimulated considerable discussion as a system to help solve the manpower shortage in our health care delivery system, and it includes many exciting possibilities. One thing for sure, AMHT in itself is not a panacea and, to be effective, it must be designed to meet a particular need. It would be disastrous to take an automated medical system predesigned for a specific purpose and attempt to apply it to all health care problems. However, I would like to describe how the Tennessee Valley Authority (TVA) has adapted our industrial medicine AMHT program to demonstrate how some of the health problems in rural areas of the Tennessee Valley might be solved.

TVA's Automated Multiphasic Health Testing System

TVA's AMHT system may be divided into four components: the automated Central Medical Laboratory, computer-processed electro-cardiograms, an automated medical information system and AMHT facilities which include a mobile health clinic and permanent medical offices.

Automated Central Medical Laboratory

The Central Medical Laboratory serves all medical facilities operated by TVA and provides support for community demonstration projects which will be discussed in more detail later. The equipment consists primarily of SMA 12 and SMA 7A AutoAnalyzers and a computer for recording data in medical records, tabulating laboratory results and

James L. Craig, M.D., M.P.H., *Medical Director, Tennessee Valley Authority, Chattanooga, Tenn.*

maintaining quality control. For input into the computer, Techniloggers with punched tape outputs are used with the SMA 12 and SMA 7A systems.

Computer Processed Electrocardiograms

TVA has been involved in computer electrocardiography since 1966, and during that time we have certainly had our ups and downs and our encouraging and disappointing moments. However, for the past two years our computer ECG program has stabilized, and although the program still has some shortcomings, we have a reliable ECG screening system. TVA utilizes its IBM computer, using Version D of the Public Health Service's program, to analyze electrocardiograms from TVA's employee health service and from several community demonstration projects.

In our experience we have found the computer to be highly useful for analyzing ECGs when most of the tracings are normal, such as in periodic examination programs. However, in our experience with hospital patients, we have found the computer to be something less than perfect (Fig. 1).

Automated Medical Information System

An automated medical information system, which has been in operation since 1966, is capable of maintaining medical records for 25,000 employees scattered over an 80,000-square-mile area. The system is also used to perform administrative tasks such as computerized medical follow-up of abnormal conditions, the storage of medical record data in easily retrievable form and preparation of administrative reports (Fig. 2).

Automated Multiphasic Health Testing Facilities

The automated regional medical laboratory, computer electrocardiography and the automated medical information system are tied together to provide automated multiphasic health testing. Initially, our AMHT program was developed as a method to provide periodic health evaluations on employees working in remote work locations, and consequently, our first experience with AMHT was on mobile clinics. Our experience with mobile clinics dates back to 1942 and our present third-generation mobile facility has been in operation since 1965. In addition to being an effective method of providing periodic health inventories on employees at remote work sites, we have found that mobile AMHT units enable health care providers to live in the city and extend their professional services to rural areas (Fig. 3).

Mobile Health Clinic

The Mobile Health Clinic visits remote work sites at approximately two-year intervals. The examination on this six-station unit includes history, height, weight, blood pressure, vision and hearing tests, computer electrocardiogram, tonometry, chest x-ray, urinalysis and blood specimens which are analyzed in the central medical laboratory.

The clinic is principally a mobile health-data collection station which is staffed by two medical technicians and one clerk. It takes approximately 20 minutes to process a screenee and the cost is approximately $35 per examination. In a usual workday, the unit is programmed to test 25 employees (Fig. 4).

Permanent Medical Offices

In addition to AMHT on our mobile unit, similar testing is also available at our permanent medical facilities in Chattanooga, Knoxville and Nashville, Tennessee, and Muscle Shoals, Alabama. Also, these area centers serve as hubs for our employee health program, with satellite nurse practitioner stations at steam plants, major medical units at construction sites, etc.

Community Demonstration Projects

Since TVA has long recognized that efforts in economic and social development must include opportunities for Valley residents to improve their health status, we have made available our employee health screening techniques to demonstrate their potential value for the public in the Tennessee Valley. The AMHT program which we have demonstrated in the rural areas of Mississippi and Appalachia differs somewhat from our employee program because the system has been adapted to meet different needs, and we paid particular attention to making the rural projects, as much as practical, a part of the region's health care delivery plan.

Northeast Mississippi Demonstrations

Our first experience in the use of mobile multiphasic health testing in rural areas was in 1968 when 500 residents of northeast Mississippi were examined in our mobile clinic. This was a cooperative project involving TVA, local medical societies, the University of Tennessee, the Regional Medical Program and the Mississippi State Board of Health. The 1,900 abnormalities detected during this demonstration convinced the eight

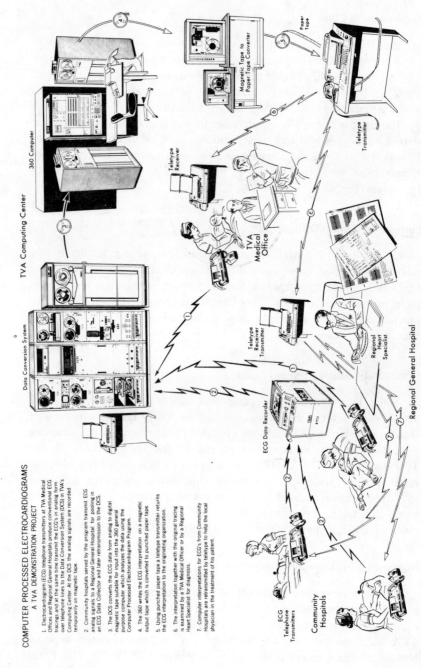

COMPUTER PROCESSED ELECTROCARDIOGRAMS
A TVA DEMONSTRATION PROJECT

1. Electrocardiogram (ECG) telephone transmitters at TVA Medical Offices and Regional General Hospitals produce conventional ECG tracings and at the same time transmit the ECG's in analog form over telephone lines to the Data Conversion System (DCS) in TVA's Computing Center. At the DCS the analog signals are recorded temporarily on magnetic tape.

2. Community hospitals served by the program transmit ECG analog signals to a Regional General Hospital for pooling in an ECG Data Collector and later retransmission to the DCS.

3. The DCS converts the ECG data from analog to digital magnetic tape suitable for input into the 360 general purpose computer which analyzes the data using the Computer Processed Electrocardiogram Program.

4. The 360 writes the ECG interpretation on a magnetic output tape which is converted to punched paper tape.

5. Using punched paper tape a teletype transmitter returns the ECG interpretation to the originating organization.

6. The interpretation together with the original tracing is examined by a TVA Medical Officer or by a Regional Heart Specialist for diagnosis.

7. Computer interpretations for ECG's from Community Hospitals are retransmitted by teletype to help the local physician in the treatment of his patient.

Figure 1.

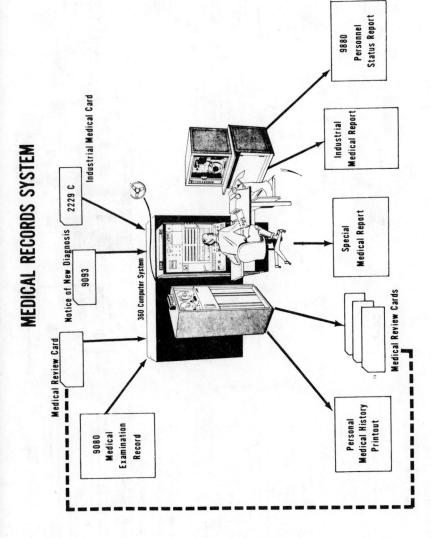

MEDICAL RECORDS SYSTEM

Medical Review Card

Notice of New Diagnosis

Industrial Medical Card

9093

2229 C

9080 Medical Examination Record

360 Computer System

9880 Personnel Status Report

Industrial Medical Report

Special Medical Report

Medical Review Cards

Personal Medical History Printout

Figure 2.

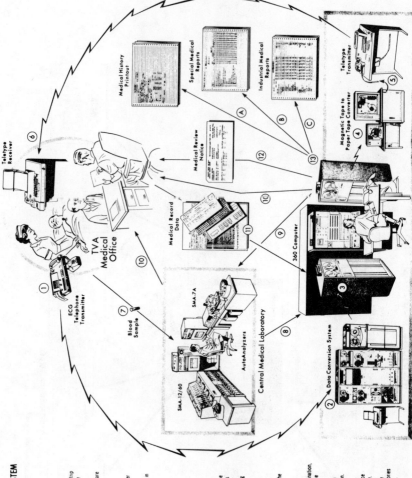

OPERATIONAL AUTOMATED MEDICAL SYSTEM
TENNESSEE VALLEY AUTHORITY
DIVISION OF MEDICAL SERVICES

ELECTROCARDIOGRAMS

1. ECG's are taken in the medical office by an ECG Telephone Transmitter, a device which both produces a conventional strip chart of the heart's action and transmits the information by telephone to the computing center.

2. The ECG's are received by the Data Conversion System and are converted into a form which can be used by the computer.

3. The computer receives and processes the ECG's.

4. The computer's analysis is converted from magnetic computer tape to punched paper tape.

5. This paper tape can be read by a teletype transmitter, which in turn sends the processed ECG back to the medical office.

6. The results are received by a teletype receiver, providing the medical office with both the original strip chart and a computer-analyzed printout for interpretation by the staff.

BLOOD ANALYSIS

7. A blood sample is taken in the medical office and sent to TVA's Central Medical Laboratory.

8. At the laboratory the blood is analyzed by the SMA-7A and the SMA-12/60 AutoAnalyzers. These units record their analyses (19 separate tests) on both punched paper tape and charts. The paper tape is sent to the computing center for processing by the computer.

9. The computer produces both individual reports and recaps of the aggregate. The recaps are sent back to the laboratory.

10. The computer printouts and the SMA charts are returned to the medical office.

MEDICAL EXAMINATION INFORMATION SYSTEM

11. When the medical office completes any kind of medical examination, the results are tabulated on special forms to be included in the computing center's medical records systems.

12. The computer automatically generates follow-up notices which were requested by the medical staff at the time of examination. The computer checks the Personnel Management Information System's master tape for the location of the employee. (TVA employees may change location frequently) and sends the notice of follow-up examination to the appropriate TVA medical facility.

13. Upon request, the computer is capable of producing almost any kind of medical report desired, from (A) individual medical histories to (B) special medical reports to (C) industrial medical reports. This system makes for a speedier, more efficient, and less cumbersome method of medical record-keeping.

Figure 3.

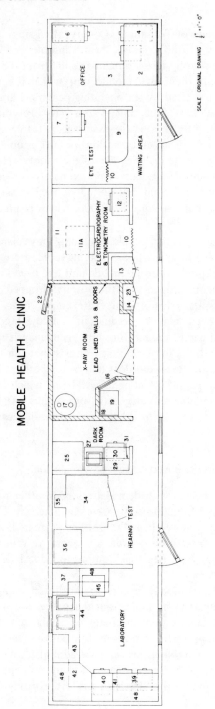

Figure 4.

practicing physicians of Tishomingo County, Mississippi, that AMHT could help solve some of the county's health problems. Subsequently, the Tishomingo County physicians obtained funds from the Regional Medical Program and built their own mobile unit which is screening 65 to 70 people daily. It is staffed by six operating personnel and is supported by six follow-up workers. The unit is open to everyone, including the physicians' private patients, and the examination is free of charge.

During the first year of operation 10,000 people received AMHT examinations. This figure includes 80% of the county's school children and 50% of all the county's residents. Approximately 60% of those screened by the unit require follow-up, but only 30% need to see a physician. The annual budget is approximately $200,000, which results in a cost of $20 per examination.

The enthusiasm of the people, including physicians, is an apparent endorsement of the program, but something more interesting has occurred at the county hospital. After the mobile unit had been in operation for six months, the patient occupancy of the hospital dropped 30%. For the first time in the hospital's history there are empty beds, and 20 hospital personnel have been laid off because of the low hospital census. The reason for this apparent reduced hospital occupancy is not entirely clear, but Dr. Harry Cosby, a local physician, insists that the AMHT unit is the only changed factor. He is confident that, among other things, multiphasic examinations give people a feeling of well-being which has resulted in less demand for hospital-based diagnostic procedures. At least, no one in Tishomingo County can say he is being denied medical care.

Demonstrations in the Poverty Areas of Appalachia

We have also helped with demonstrations in other rural areas. During the summer of 1970, 6,200 people were examined by TVA's multiphasic health facility and more than 4,000 were examined during a six-week project in 1971. These projects were a cooperative venture by Vanderbilt University, Appalachian Regional Commission, local health departments and TVA.

TVA provided its mobile multiphasic health screening clinic, technical assistance and supervision, and automated processing of medical laboratory tests. The students were in charge of regular scheduling, examining and providing appropriate follow-up for persons screened during the "Health Fairs." Vanderbilt University was administratively responsible for the project and faculty members supervised the students. Local residents played an active role in the "Health Fairs" by assisting in the nonprofessional activities.

These rural projects demonstrated that mobile multiphasic health testing can be effective in identifying people in need of health care; raising the standard of health care for people already under some form of medical treatment by providing diagnostic studies previously unavailable in their communities; and expanding a medical school campus to include a different population group, thereby allowing students to examine and gain experience from patients other than those found in the metropolitan clinic.

To date, the local accomplishments of the Appalachia AMHT projects include the establishment of locally operated nursing clinics in White Oak, Briceville and Deer Lodge, Tennessee, and improvement in the services provided by a previously established nursing clinic in Clairfield, Tennessee.

Accomplishments at Vanderbilt University include the establishment of a nurse practitioner program with the first students coming from nurses who participated in the Appalachia project, the establishment of a center for community health services which is pledged to study methods of improving health care in rural areas, and assignment of a medical intern to spend six months of his internship in rural Appalachia working under the supervision of the Vanderbilt Medical School faculty.

Listing these accomplishments does not imply that we have found the solution to the health problems of rural Appalachia. There are many social and economic ills which significantly interfere with attempts to improve the health of the people, although mobile multiphasic health testing is effective in providing diagnostic services previously unavailable and in identifying many health problems which need consultation and therapeutic attention.

We found, particularly in the Appalachian areas, that the economics of medical care is often a significant deterrent to the provision of many therapeutic services. Economic factors keep surrounding communities from accepting indigent, out-of-county residents except under emergency circumstances. Consequently, it is most difficult to obtain routine hospital services for the poor, and the major treatment successes in the health fairs were for those conditions that could be handled on an emergency or out-patient basis. Although the health departments are quite sympathetic with the needs of the people and support the health screening project, they have neither the funds nor the commitment at this time to accept the responsibility for obtaining needed hospital care.

I am not implying that there is a lack of good faith in attempts to meet the identified health needs of our rural citizens. I am just pointing out a realistic fact: Social and economic developments have not kept pace with developments in medical science which already has produced the techniques to provide better health care delivery for all the people who desire health care.

Summary

TVA's experience in occupational medicine AMHT has demonstrated that multiphasic health testing can be effective in providing periodic health inventories and in forming the nucleus of a systemized health care delivery plan for people of all income levels. For rural populations, mobile multiphasic health testing has been demonstrated to be a method of improving medical care by serving as a point of entry into the health care system and by raising the level of medical care through expanded diagnostic services in rural communities.

The problems of medical manpower shortage in rural areas may find a partial answer in techniques such as mobile multiphasic health testing and computerized processes which allow physicians to live in the city and at the same time extend their services to rural areas. It is imperative that these techniques and programs be developed in conjunction with and supported by comprehensive health care delivery concepts which include social and economic considerations.

Objective Measurements of Early Vascular Disease

Robert D. Allison

Introduction

Arterial vascular pathological changes frequently precede the development of clinical signs and symptoms, and it is important to detect the "silent changes" quantitatively and correlate the findings with other clinical data. Systemic hypertension and arterial vascular obstructive disease can be evaluated at an early stage and documented through systematic use of vascular laboratory diagnostic procedures. All tests to be described are conducted in a constant temperature (25°C) and constant humidity (40%) environment. All vasoactive drugs are withheld for 48 hours prior to the procedures, and subjects are requested to refrain from smoking for at least two hours before the test procedures.

The Cold Pressor Test (Fig. 1)

Following basal blood pressure measurement, one of the patient's hands (up to the wrist) is immersed in cold water (4°C) for one minute while the blood pressure of the opposite arm is recorded every 15 seconds. Normally, this stimulus produces a rise in blood pressure of less than 25 mm of mercury, systolic and 15 mm of mercury, diastolic. As soon as the blood pressure has returned to the base level, the procedure is repeated on the opposite hand. Patients who are hyper-reactors are characterized by marked increases in systolic and diastolic pressure in response to the cold water stress. The tendency for hyper-reactors to develop sustained hypertension in later life has been well documented.

The Cold Immersion Test (Fig. 2)

Mercury strain gauges are placed on fingers and pulse tracings are taken immediately before and 5, 10 and 15 minutes after immersion of the hand in cold water (4°C) for one minute. The healthy subject is characterized

---

Robert D. Allison, Ph.D., *Scott and White Clinic, Temple, Tex.*

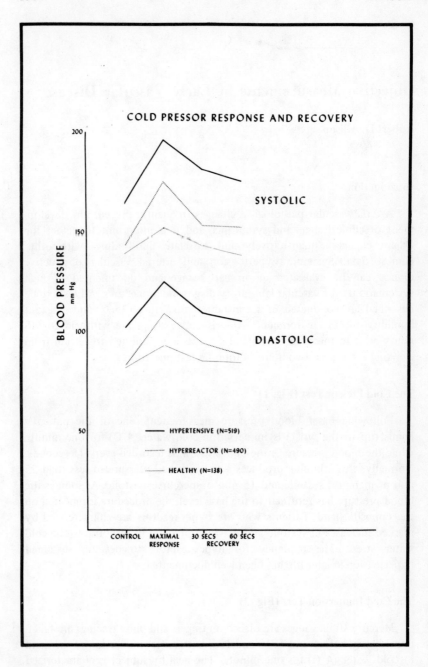

Figure 1.

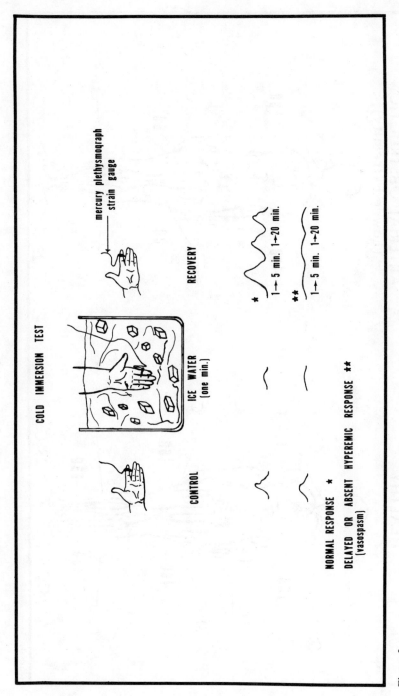

Figure 2.

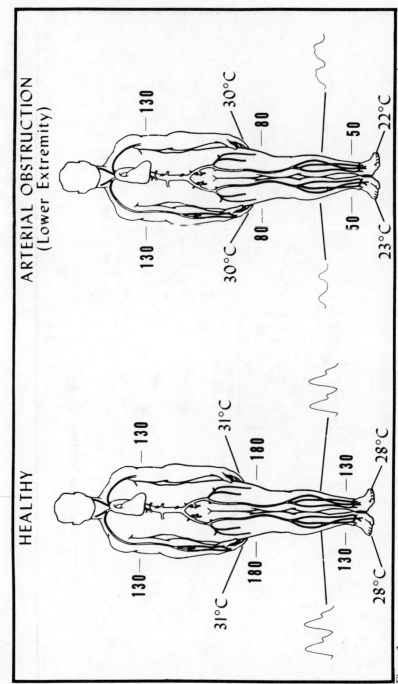

Figure 3.

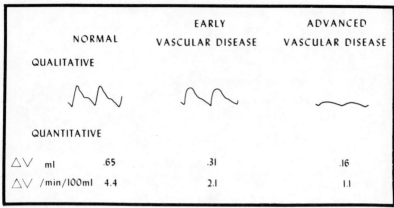

Figure 4.

by a hyperemic response and an increase in recorded pulse amplitude within 10-15 minutes compared with recorded control pulse amplitudes. Patients with vasospasm are characterized by a delayed hyperemia and exaggerated vasoconstriction, often persisting for greater than 15 minutes. This test is useful for assessing vasospastic conditions and is helpful in detecting Raynaud's disease.

Skin Temperatures, Pressure Gradients and Calf Blood Flow (Fig. 3)

The systematic use of skin temperature measurements of fingers and toes, mercury plethysmographic measurements of the pressure gradients between the upper and lower extremity and impedance plethysmographic measurements of blood pulse volume and blood flow to calf segments has provided a simple and nontraumatic appraisal of early arterial vascular disease and hypertensive processes. Normal blood flow values for healthy calf segments have been established for large populations of subjects in a broad age category, and abnormal blood flow values have been correlated with clinical and radiological evidence.

Contour Analysis of Calf Pulse Curves (Fig. 4)

Contour analysis of pulse curves recorded from calf segments (impedance plethysmography) provides definitive information concerning physiological vasoconstriction responses, the vasospasm associated with asymptomatic vascular pathology and the presence of major arterial obstructive disease with or without evidence of collateral circulation.

Coronary Profile: Ethical Considerations

William B. Kannel

Vascular diseases of the heart and brain constitute the leading cause of death and account for a considerable amount of disability in the elderly. Treatment and rehabilitation of the completed catastrophe is obviously less rewarding than its prevention. However, atherosclerosis, the anatomical basis for about half the deaths in the western world, has thus far resisted efforts recommended for either its cure or prevention. The appalling annual toll of cardiovascular mortality continues unabated.

Because of the natural history of these diseases, it has become apparent that only a preventive approach offers the possibility of achieving a substantial reduction in coronary and stroke mortality.[1] Prevention requires knowledge of the factors which predispose. Strokes are not an accident of nature as the term "vascular accident" implies and coronary attacks are not an inevitable consequence of aging; each is rather the end result of a chain of host and environmental circumstances evolving over decades. Many kinds of evidence suggest that environmental factors exert a large influence on the incidence of coronary disease. An understanding of these mechanisms is the strategic goal in research in this field because it is presumed that out of this some preventive modifications through environmental control could come.

Epidemiologic investigations of the way coronary attacks and strokes arise and evolve in general population samples in Framingham and elsewhere have begun to identify highly vulnerable persons and the factors which predispose.[2,3] Estimates of the risk associated with identified precursors of these atherosclerotic diseases have been ascertained. The major risk factors thus far identified include hypercholesterolemia, hypertension, impaired carbohydrate tolerance, ECG abnormalities, obesity, the cigarette habit and lack of physical exercise.[4-10] Using some of these variables, it is possible to compute an atherogenic profile for asymptomatic persons in the general population which allows estimation of the probability of developing a coronary or cerebral vascular attack over

William B. Kannel, M.D., *Medical Director, National Institute of Health, Heart Disease Epidemiology Study, Framingham, Mass.*

a wide range. With the advent of automated laboratory procedures, the technology required to identify vulnerable persons and to estimate their risk of an attack requires nothing more than a simple blood sample; a static and postexercise ECG; and determination of the blood pressure, body weight and cigarette habit. Large segments of the population can be rapidly and efficiently screened if desired.

Size and Nature of the Problem

The magnitude of the problem of cardiovascular disease hardly needs emphasis since it is the leading cause of premature death.[1] Brain infarction and progressive deterioration, the usual course of hypertensive myocardial failure,[1,2] will have to be conquered by timely, effective and sustained intervention, implemented to control multiple contributors to their occurrence identified in asymptomatic persons as early in life as possible.

Coronary disease, the leading cardiovascular killer, is a disease which characteristically strikes with little warning, in which the first symptom is often sudden death and in which more than half the mortality occurs outside the hospital in a matter of minutes.[1] It can be silent even in its most dangerous form; one in four myocardial infarctions goes unrecognized.[11]

Proof of Efficacy

It must be admitted that there is no secure basis for estimating the reduction in coronary morbidity and mortality that might be expected from correction of risk factors. Data from Framingham would suggest that correction of four common risk factors in young men – overweight, hypercholesterolemia, hypertension and the cigarette habit – might reduce their coronary incidence quite substantially (Table 1). However, converting a person from a high- to a low-risk status is not necessarily equivalent to always having had low-risk attributes.

The evidence from field and clinical trials that lowering high blood pressure and high cholesterol levels results in improved coronary disease rates is still equivocal.[12-14] The benefits of reducing overweight, while it does reduce blood pressure and blood lipids and improve carbohydrate tolerance (as regards cardiovascular mortality), are based only on possibly biased life insurance data.[10,15] Correction of impaired glucose tolerance has not yet been shown to lower cardiovascular mortality; indeed, some claim certain hypoglycemic agents produce higher death rates.[16] Evidence that altering the composition of the diet to lower blood lipid values results in a lowering of coronary risk is still disputed, although most accept the A.H.A. dietary recommendations as sound.[17] There is no evidence to

TABLE 1. Twelve-Year Risk of Coronary Disease for Differing Levels
of Risk Factor — Framingham Men, 1948-1960

Serum Cholesterol Value	Systolic Blood Pressure	Relative Weight	Cigarette Smoking	New Events Per 1000		
				Age 35	45	55
250	150	110	1 pkg.	67	209	261
220	150	110	1 pkg.	35	175	212
220	130	110	1 pkg.	23	152	164
220	130	100	1 pkg.	20	120	154
220	130	100	0 pkg.	6	54	95

Age Group at Exam 1:

30-39 $y = \log_e [P/(1-P)] = -17.6 + 0.023_{x_1} + 0.022_{x_2} + 0.032_{x_3} + 0.598_{x_4} + 0.092_{x_5}$

40-49 $y = \log_e [P/(1-P)] = -13.7 + 0.007_{x_1} + 0.009_{x_2} + 0.027_{x_3} + 0.434_{x_4} + 0.120_{x_5}$

50-62 $y = \log_e [P/(1-P)] = -11.1 + 0.009_{x_1} + 0.016_{x_2} + 0.008_{x_3} + 0.272_{x_4} + 0.072_{x_5}$

From: Cornfield, J. and Mitchell, S.: Selected Risk Factors in Coronary Disease. *Arch. Environ. Health,* 19:382-394, 1969.

prove that physical exercise improves the risk of sedentary persons or revascularizes their myocardium by promoting collaterals. There is evidence that cessation of cigarette smoking improves the coronary mortality rate since ex-smokers have been demonstrated to have a substantially lower risk than those who continue to smoke,[9] but no rigorously designed field trials are available to unequivocally corroborate this.

Nevertheless, the potential for salvage of coronary-vulnerable persons by such measures is great, the hazard small, and the rewards include other benefits in addition to coronary prevention. If the therapy of existing cardiovascular disease were put to the same rigorous tests of efficacy, i.e., that it delays recurrences and prolongs life, we might be reduced to therapeutic nihilism. However the need to do something for persons with symptoms — even if not of proven efficacy — seems easier to justify.

Coping with Risk Factors

While a scientific theory and justification for coronary prophylaxis may exist, the means for coping with coronary precursors is in a primitive state compared to methodology for assessing risk. Additional research to find effective methods for safely correcting risk factors without causing too much disruption in established living patterns is required. The general hygienic measures indicated (curbing the cigarette habit, taking more exercise, reducing overweight and dieting) are not easy to implement. Our record for achieving sustained weight reduction in the obese for long periods is not good, but gaining adherence to any kind of dietary restriction has always been a difficult enterprise. Nor do we know how to get the habituated heavy cigarette smoker to give up the habit. Most individuals find it is difficult to take an adequate amount of exercise. Also, we do not know the optimal exercise prescription for a sedentary, flabby, middle-aged, coronary-prone subject. We do not have enough trained personnel to supervise exercise in such persons so that they do not execute themselves by precipitous overindulgence. Also, a life-long dependence on medicines to control blood pressure, blood cholesterol and blood sugar is not without expense or potential hazard. In any event, it is difficult to gain adherence to long-term prophylactic drug regimens in asymptomatic persons. Good health education, an enthusiastic physician and frequent periodic checks for adherence, efficacy and side effects are crucial to the success of such an endeavor.

The prevention of cardiovascular disease involves attention to what many physicians often regard as medical trivia. Because of the large number of susceptibles involved, it will be necessary to find additional qualified personnel willing and able to implement and supervise the prophylactic program. Better methods will have to be found for coping with identified risk factors. Proof of efficacy will have to be sought to convince the subject and the physician that a sustained effort is worthwhile. The value of detecting occult medical impairments leading to cardiovascular disease depends not only on our ability to identify them or on their economic and medical importance as forces of mortality, but also on the availability of resources for effectively coping with them and evidence that this will result in substantial benefit to all engaged in the endeavor.

Preventive trials in chronic disease deserve a high priority. A substantial reduction in the annual toll of cardiovascular mortality will require considerable change in attitudes, behavior, sociocultural attributes, economics and a more favorable balancing of the ecology. Multifactor preventive intervention is more likely to succeed than that restricted to a single precursor. Risk is compounded by multiple factors and it is difficult to modify single factors without, at the same time, altering others. Thus, logic dictates an attempt to simultaneously modify the major risk factors.

Yield: Prevention of Public Health

Theoretically, with modern computerized, automated technology, we now have the capability for seeking out of the general population persons with early asymptomatic cardiovascular disease and those at increased risk of acquiring it. However, there are difficult logistic problems to be solved.

The high prevalence of risk factors in the general population and the proportion of the coronary incidence that arises from various categories of risk poses problems. Those in the upper decile of risk, as determined by their "coronary profile," have at least 10 times the risk of those in the lowest decile, but only 20% of the total burden of disease arises out of this high-risk group. A coronary profile can, however, select those in gravest danger. Also, such persons can be more readily motivated to follow a prophylactic regimen, and their physicians can be more easily convinced of the urgency to implement the indicated measure.

On the other hand, approximately 80% of the male U.S. population has one or more risk factors and out of this huge reservoir some 90% of the coronary disease evolves. Successful intervention in this group should make a major impact on coronary mortality. However, to screen the entire population periodically and place those identified by this criterion under prophylactic medical management would seem impractical. What emerges then is the conclusion that the entire population must be regarded as vulnerable and in need of alteration of the living habits which appear to be promoting cardiovascular disease. This entails a broad, public health approach involving environmental control to remove cardiovascular "pollutants." Detecting and coping with identified cardiovascular disease precursors is often beyond the capability of the potential victim and his physician, overwhelmed in discharging his obligation to those already ill. Thus, it is properly a community concern since these diseases constitute a considerable burden to the community in loss of expert manpower, drain on medical resources and welfare funds.

Because of the broad scope of the changes required for the general population, the difficulties in implementing them and the remaining uncertainties about efficacy, we are restricted to a preventive medicine approach which focuses attention on highly vulnerable persons identified either through periodic screening or by the physician during periodic office visits. Despite the relative popularity of screening, periodic health evaluation and the concept of disease prevention, preventive medicine clinics in this country are few in number. Patients must be motiviated to undertake and follow a life-long program of prophylaxis with periodic reevaluation for acquisition of new risk factors, success in controlling old ones and the appearance of early evidence of asymptomatic cardiovascular disease. Both the potential coronary candidate and his physician will require considerable assistance in their collaborative venture. This will require a concerted effort involving voluntary health agencies, public health agencies and health insurance groups. To embark on such an endeavor without a better understanding of how to ensure adherence is likely to provide a frustrating experience for all concerned. However, endeavors to detect and correct contributors to cardiovascular disease should stimulate discoveries concerning the natural history of the presymptomatic stage of the disease, create new drugs and instruments and major improvements in the way to correct and cope with disease precursors.

Nature of Periodic Health Evaluation

It is difficult to delineate with any assurance the boundaries between automated multiphasic screening and comprehensive annual health check-ups. Screening implies a more rapid and superficial assessment employing fewer definitive diagnostic procedures, designed to sort out large numbers of people into those who are and are not medically impaired. This must be done while the condition is still asymptomatic and must detect abnormalities not already known to the subject. To be worthwhile, the impairments detected must be important contributors to disease and there must be evidence that they can be corrected with benefit to the subject.

"Screening" for asymptomatic coronary disease or its precursors can be done, using modern technology, in such a way as to provide definitive diagnostic information or a reasonably precise, comprehensive coronary profile. Blood can be processed in an automated laboratory and this information, along with a computer-read ECG, blood pressure, automated history information and other findings, fed into a computer. A coronary risk profile can then be computed and available before the subject leaves the premises. The subject can be immediately plugged into the medical care delivery system for prophylactic management without undergoing further diagnostic procedures.

Computers can also be programmed to compare information with acceptable assigned ranges of "normal" or optimal values. A medical report of the "abnormality" can then be printed out along with the recommended next procedure, medical disposition, provisional diagnosis, computed coronary profile and management recommendations. Copies of medical reports can be sent to the private physician and retained by the screener for comparison with subsequent follow-up evaluation. Subsequent appointments and follow-up inquiries can be made automatically with standard IBM techniques used for billing delinquencies.

Hazards to the Potential Beneficiary

In addition to potential benefits, there are also hazards to screening for previously unknown health impairments or presymptomatic precursors of lethal disease. Being placed under medical management can be costly, dangerous, psychologically disquieting, and disruptive of one's life style. However, those with complaints may be falsely reassured by a periodic health examination not specifically designed to investigate their particular discomfort. Iatrogenic illness may be created by preliminary screening abnormalities not confirmed by later tests, making the subject overly concerned with some "laboratory illness." Unless properly carried out, there may be an assault on the sense of security and generation of unwarranted apprehension.

Mechanisms to facilitate automation of health data could very well lead to networks for processing which might include national, state and local medical societies, hospital and university medical centers, insurance carriers, government claims facilities and others with a legitimate interest in medical and health data. The potential for both good and evil is great.

The medical profession has an important duty to guide the development of computer storage and retrieval systems for personal medical information to protect the privileged communication between the patient and his physician. This is essential if the confidence and integrity of the physician-patient relationship is to be maintained.

There is little doubt that efficient, economical means for precise health evaluation can be devised. Health maintenance organizations are being promoted by the present administration. Thus, the issue of periodic health evaluation has assumed increased relevance and immediacy. It seems inevitable that such endeavors will eventually come under some degree of government regulation since competition and economic incentives alone cannot be relied upon to prevent abuses. Such regulation also affects the way medical services are delivered.

Properly used, periodic health evaluation should be a valuable tool in preventive medicine and should provide entry into the medical care delivery system at a point in the course of illness when more effective intervention can be accomplished. At the very least, screening programs could find chronic illness previously undetected and ensure that those most significant get priority for treatment. Periodic health evaluation makes possible the diagnosis and management of chronic disease before it reaches an irreversible stage, allowing greater possibility for improvement. This stage of chronic illness, at present, often goes undetected. These possible benefits must be weighed against the hazards and uncertainties.

The hope is that, in the long run, periodic screening will greatly reduce medical costs but there is at present no assurance that this is the case. Periodic health evaluations to detect presymptomatic conditions can hasten this transition and provide better care at a lower cost. However, we must demonstrate that the costs to the community are commensurate with the benefits. Overutilization and duplication must be avoided. The endeavor must not compete with therapeutic medicine for resources in short supply; it must be either integrated into the system, utilizing resources more efficiently, or it must provide its own services and personnel. The sick must still be given high priority in the competition for medical resources. The beneficiary of periodic health evaluation must not be deprived of quality care when he becomes ill.

Implications for the Physician

Automation, involving computers, can be justified only if it allows care to be provided economically and gives the physician more time to spend with patients. The quality as well as the quantity of care provided must be improved, both at lower cost.

Physician group practices, industrial medical establishments, insurance companies, labor organizations and the like will be called upon to provide the service. This moves a large segment of medical care away from the individual private practitioner and the fee-for-service arrangement, a system of care not to be lightly dismissed. This makes for less personalized care. The patient no longer has the attention of his own physician, directly compensated for his efforts in his patient's behalf, and is forced into group and third-party arrangements.

Under the system of therapeutic medicine, the responsibility of the physician is restricted to patients who seek his services and the initiative of the patient is required to gain entry into the medical care delivery system. Health maintenance endeavors place on the physician the responsibility for bringing medical resources to bear, although the subject must still present himself for the screening or periodic health examination. The *modus operandi* of the physician is thus changed from a solo endeavor to one in close collaboration with divers auxiliary medical personnel. The physician now must practice in a group in some sort of community health center with modern medical technology and data processing at his disposal. He must acclimatize and learn how to use these effectively. If health maintenance is to be delivered on a mass scale, it is probably not desirable to divert the physician directly to this task. He can only be expected to direct or supervise the endeavor. Allied health personnel will have to be trained not only to perform the periodic health evaluation but to participate in implementing the appropriate corrective measures. The subject or beneficiary of this endeavor must be willing to accept care from such nonprofessional personnel. Further, preventive medical findings will have to be shared with the patient. The patient will be required to be a much more active partner in his own health care.

The attitude of the physician is a major stumbling block to effective coronary prophylaxis. The prevention of cardiovascular disease involves attention to what he often regards as "medical trivia." The physician must come to regard the occurrence of strokes, coronary heart disease and congestive heart failure in persons under medical surveillance as medical failures rather than the point at which he initiates medical management. Also, he feels less comfortable prescribing hygienic measures than medicines and ineffectual dispensing advice such as can be obtained from *Reader's Digest* and would rather prescribe a pill to counteract faulty living habits.

It seems clear that the present health care delivery system is unable to cope adequately with the large load of illness presented to it. It is not geared for health maintenance or preventive medicine and responds largely to the urgent demands of life-threatening medical crises. When a periodic health evaluation and preventive maintenance program is developed, people will be given the choice between fee-for-service, item-by-item and prepayment or both. Per capita and fee-for-service approaches are not mutually exclusive and both can be run through the same system. Current third-party payment mechanisms, as regards health maintenance, tend to be overly responsive to in-patient care and too therapeutically oriented. A per capita system allows for and may encourage the laboratory tests and out-patient periodic examinations essential to a prevention-oriented system. The physician and patient would, however, be required to adapt to this less personalized type of medical care.

Most physicians are puzzled and uneasy about the changes taking place in concepts of medical care. Early detection and presymptomatic diagnosis and management of disease involves a change in the technology and philosophy of medicine. The physician will require a period of reorientation before he can contend with the new concepts. This way of practicing must be made attractive to large numbers of physicians and acceptable to patients. The physician must be kept free of bureaucratic constraints on professional judgment essential to the practice of good medicine. New organizations will be needed, freed from older patterns of clinical practice and thinking, which will employ advanced techniques of industry and scientific management. Active opposition of some clinicians can be anticipated. Unless the enthusiastic support of the bulk of the medical profession for these concepts is won, there is little likelihood of the endeavor's gaining acceptance and wide application and less of its succeeding in its objectives.

References

1. Gordon, T., Kannel, W. B.: Premature mortality from coronary heart disease: The Framingham Study. *JAMA*, 215:1617-1625, 1971.
2. Kannel, W. B.: Current status of the epidemiology of brain infarction associated with occlusive arterial disease. *Stroke*, 2:295-318, 1971.
3. Kannel, W. B., McNamara, P.: The evidence for excess risk in coronary heart disease. *Minnesota Med.*, 52:1197-1201, 1969.

4. Doyle, J. T., Heslin, A. S., Hilleboe, H. E., et al.: Early diagnosis of ischemic heart disease. *New Eng. J. Med.*, 261:1096-1101, 1959.

5. Kannel, W. B., Gordon, T., Sorlie, P., et al.: Physical activity and coronary vulnerability: The Framingham Study. *Cardiol. Digest*, 6:28-40, 1971.

6. Kannel, W. B., Gordon, T., Castelli, W. P., et al.: Electrocardiographic left ventricular hypertrophy and risk of coronary heart disease: The Framingham Study. *Ann. Int. Med.*, 72:813-822, 1970.

7. Kannel, W. B., Castelli, W. P., Gordon, T., et al.: Serum cholesterol, lipoproteins and risk of coronary heart disease: The Framingham Study. *Ann. Int. Med.*, 74:1-12, 1971.

8. Kannel, W. B., Gordon, T., and Schwartz, M. J.: Systolic versus diastolic blood pressure and risk of coronary heart disease: The Framingham Study. *Amer. J. Cardiol.*, 27:335-346, 1971.

9. Kannel, W. B., Castelli, W. P., and McNamara, P. M.:*Cigarette Smoking and Risk of Coronary Heart Disease: Epidemiologic Clues to Pathogenesis, The Framingham Study.* National Cancer Institute, Monograph No. 28, 1968.

10. Kannel, W. B., LeBauer, E. J., Dawber, T. R., et al.: Relation of body weight to development of coronary heart disease: The Framingham Study. *Circulation*, 35:734-744, 1967.

11. Kannel, W. B., McNamara, P. M., Feinleib, M., et al.: The unrecognized myocardial infarction. Fourteen year follow-up experience in the Framingham Study. *Geriatrics*, 25:75-87, 1970.

12. Freis, E. D.: VA cooperative study group on anti-hypertensive agents. Effects of treatment on morbidity in hypertension. *JAMA*, 202:1028, 1967 and *JAMA*, 213:1143, 1970.

13. Leren, P.: The effect of plasma cholesterol lowering diet in male survivors of myocardial infarction. *Acta Med. Scand.* (suppl.) 466:1-92, 1966.

14. Dayton, S., Pearce, M. L., Hashimoto, S. et al.: A controlled clinical trial of a diet high in unsaturated fat in preventing complications of atherosclerosis. *Circulation*, 40:(suppl. II):1-63, 1969.

15. Marks, H. H.: Influence of obesity on morbidity and mortality. *Bull. N.Y. Acad. Med.*, 36:296, 1960.

16. University Group Diabetes Program. A study of the effects of hypoglycemic agents on vascular complications in patients with adult-onset diabetes. Part I. Design methods and baseline characteristics. Part II. Mortality results. *Diabetes,* 19(suppl. II):747-830, 1970.

17. Kannel, W. B.: The disease of living. *Nutrition Today* 6:2-11, 1971.

Report Form of the Automated ECG From Considerations for Acceptability and Efficiency

Russell L. Sandberg

Reports from automated screening should be short, neat and pertinent, since remote communications are often needed; unnecessary words are also a needless expense. A final consideration is the design of the copy producing machine itself and improper format may cause an increase in machine failure. An example demonstrating these principles is the report form commonly in use with automated electrocardiograms (Fig. 1).

To the uninitiated, this report is impressive but unintelligible. The large table of numbers suggests complicated and powerful arithmetic at work. The diagnostic statements are typically dwarfed by the table of measurements. It does not take long to perceive that these numbers are sometimes inaccurate and of dubious utility to the clinician.

The report does resemble a conventional analytic report to some extent. After seaching a 48-member table, the rate, P-R and Q-T intervals can be found. However, there are up to 12 measurements presented. These are typically different from lead to lead. A variety of angular measurements are also presented. Our experience with this form was that the clinician learned to find the patient's number and the statements of diagnostic information. All other information was ignored. This was disheartening.

A short form of this report was available as an option, but it did not include the standard interval measurements. The clinician viewed the report as incomplete.

An additional difficulty was the high cost of sending a report by teletype over long distance lines. The original form required 6 minutes. This cost was between $1.50 and $2.00. One user installed at his expense an auto-answer teletype for the express purpose of receiving the reports at night. This avoided an hour of pounding and dinging generated by the reports of 10 electrocardiograms.

A final irritant was the tendency of the Model 33 teletype to stick at the left margin if its first command was to indent.

Russell L. Sandberg, M.D., *Division of Cardiology, University of Missouri Medical Center, Columbia, Mo.*

R. L. SANDBERG

```
                    MO.RMP-EKG PROJECT-UNIVERSITY OF MO. COLUMBIA
                       COMPUTER PROCESSED ELECTROCARDIOGRAM
                                   U.M.M.C.

PT 1319558 TAPE 720 DATE 08-11-70 11:14 AM  JULIAN 262   S.S.N. 139172998
17 YR FEMALE 5 FT  2 IN  139 LBS MEDS UNKNOWN             BP UNKNOWN
---------------------------------------------------------------------------
        I     II    III   AVR   AVL   AVF    V1    V2    V3    V4    V5    V6
---------------------------------------------------------------------------
PA    .17   .14  -.05  -.11   .09   .05   .06   .13   .14   .12   .11   .10  PA
PD    .15   .07   .10   .05   .10   .05   .05   .10   .08   .07   .08   .07  PD
PPA     .     .     .     .     .  -.03     .     .     .     .     .  -.06  PPA
PPD     .     .     .     .     .   .08     .     .     .     .     .   .02  PPD
Q/SA -.04     .     .  -.76     .     .     .     .     .     .  -.09     .  Q/SA
Q/SD  .02     .     .   .04     .     .     .     .     .     .   .02     .  Q/SD
RA    .71   .79   .07   .15   .34   .43   .14   .34   .32  1.01  1.56  1.27  RA
RD    .04   .05   .02   .02   .04   .05   .02   .02   .03   .06   .04   .05  RD
SA   -.11  -.13  -.16     .  -.05  -.13 -1.01 -1.44  -.78  -.28  -.13  -.06  SA
SD    .02   .02   .02     .   .01   .02   .04   .06   .06   .02   .01   .01  SD
RPA     .     .   .04     .     .     .     .     .     .     .     .     .  RPA
RPD     .     .   .04     .     .     .     .     .     .     .     .     .  RPD
STO   .04   .03  -.03  -.03   .06     .  -.06   .05   .06   .07   .08   .10  STO
STM   .02   .01  -.02  -.04   .05  -.02   .03   .08   .12   .07   .04   .08  STM
STE   .05   .02  -.02  -.05   .06  -.02   .05   .11   .17   .09   .05   .09  STE
TA    .20   .10  -.12  -.16   .18   .05  -.11   .20   .29   .16   .13   .19  TA
---------------------------------------------------------------------------
PR    .17   .16   .17   .16   .18   .15   .16   .15   .16   .16   .13   .16  PR
QRS   .08   .07   .08   .06   .05   .07   .06   .08   .09   .08   .07   .06  QRS
QT    .46   .40   .41   .39   .42   .51   .42   .36   .39   .35   .45   .40  QT
RATE   62    69    64    68    66    76    65    68    64    63    65    70  RATE
---------------------------------------------------------------------------
CODE    2     3    2L     2     3     3     3     2     3     2     3     4  CODE
CAL    95    95    95    95    95    95    95    95    95    95    95    95  CAL
---------------------------------------------------------------------------
AXIS IN   P    QRS    T    Q    R     S   STO              ST-T  QRS-T
DEGREES  20    39  -06        36  -79  -16                   10    45
---------------------------------------------------------------------------

                                              .
                                              . NORMAL ECG
                                              .
              MSDL APPROVED VERSION           .          ------------- M.D.
                D  41-42-25-11                . AUDIO M.C. TEL NO. 314-449-XXXX
```

Figure 1.

On all counts, the report form had to be modified. To see what might be more suitable, it was useful to ask what message the report conveyed.

To an administrator or programmer operating an automated system, the report conveyed the significant content of quality control information. Even without graphic data, troubles in the processing system could be spotted from the report. It was hard to escape the conclusion that the report was designed for the persons who indeed found it useful rather than for the clinicians, who did not. Thus, the automated ECG required two quite different reports: one for the patient's physician and one for persons responsible for systems quality control. For quality control, we saw no reason to change the report. When prepared on a local printer, a large report is still inexpensive. Something quite different was needed for the physician's report.

In a system under pressure to achieve low cost and self-sufficiency, both acceptance and dollar costs must be considered. A review of customary reporting styles and a poll of physicians at our hospital showed a preference for brevity and established order. This, of course, argued well for low cost.

When stripped of the main measurement tables, clarity and orientation were notably improved even among those initiated in decoding the previous (long) form. Teletype transmission time fell from 6 minutes to 2 minutes. The smaller table of P, QRS, T and rate figures was left unchanged.

A number of questions then arose as to why the clinician had to choose the numbers which truly represented the intervals and rate. A program weakness had been unmasked by this new format. The program itself possessed no basis for discrimination.

Nonetheless, other improvements were possible. Left justification was used in every place where speed could be gained. The name of the test, patient's number, etc. were reorganized in this way. The "advertising" was moved to the bottom of the report and left-justified. The classification statement remained in its customary position at some sacrifice of speed on the basis of convention.

A number of dashes and other artwork were removed and replaced with blank spaces where these could be introduced horizontally with a single spacing command. We found that order and clarity could be obtained just as well by this means. The time-saving was appreciable. To deal with the remaining table problem, a statistical routine was devised to make a single (best) guess. Thus, single values were printed for P-R, QRS and Q-T durations. The rate was described by three numbers in customary fashion (the range and average). These choices proved quite useful to the interval program for use in the sharpening of diagnostic statements based on those measurements.

The typical report contains 3.5 diagnostic statements. Revised as described, the report not only gained speed, clarity, utility and economy, but also made possible a combination of graphic tracings and reports within one 8½ X 11 inch page.

Very few reports were too large and then only the advertising was lost. Such a report bears a striking resemblance to an ordinary hospital ECG report. It is easily photocopied. Measurements of two reviewers confirmed our impression that high reading speed was attained with this format (four times faster than with graphic data along). On review, corrections consisted mainly in striking out lines — a mechanically efficient procedure.

The new report could be teletype transmitted in an average time of 52 seconds.

We have tried mounting the report both above and below the graphics. The first method aids in rapid patient identification and reading of statements but requires many movements of the hand because the act of writing obscures the graphics. One also tends to deface the pressure-sensitive paper.

Mounting the graphics above the report makes the reviewer's job easier but sacrifices clarity for the patient's physician. Any suggestions for improvement in layout would be welcomed since few electrocardiographers find joy in reviewing large stacks of electrocardiograms.

At present, the format is well received (Fig. 2). It says preliminary report, computer processed ECG, which hospital and which patient are addressed, and what clinical information there is. Criteria are printed at the left, diagnosis at the right and, finally, a statement of diagnostic class. Below these are intervals and rate followed by angular measures.

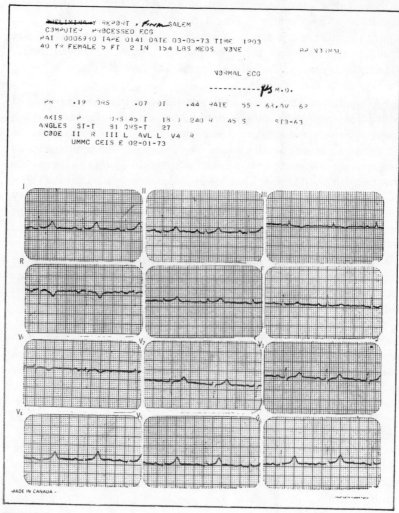

Figure 2.

Advertising comes last and no special box is provided for the physician's signature; his task includes striking out the word preliminary and signing his name.

We felt quite proud at this point at having improved acceptance and having saved time and money for all. Then we became acquainted with facsimile transmission.

One problem faced by service organizations is competition. As a university, our charter directs us to improve service and delivery of health care, but we need the goodwill of all sectors. Also, our staff is quite small and under a heavy load of teaching and patient care; no one relished reviewing an additional 200 electrocardiograms per day. Why could we not enlist the practicing cardiologist in the reviewing process by photo-facsimile? Four cardiologists in three cities were, therefore, enlisted, all more than 100 miles from the processing center and 50 miles or more from the rural hospitals they served. By photofacsimile transmission made possible by the new report form, we transmitted the graphic information and the computer report for their review.

This method was an apparent success, but one old problem returned. Of all the machinery initially tested, none would transmit the graphic data with sufficient quality in less than 6 minutes. We were again in the clutches of the telephone company. One of the facsimile companies provided the needed breakthrough for 3-minute transmission. This lowered telephone costs to $.75 per ECG. A computer plotter was necessary to maintain the resolution using 3-minute transmission. Still, a flaw in this very attractive method is the speed of facsimile transmission. A 3-minute transmission system gives favorable transmission results. It remains for a successful 1-minute transmitter to produce genuine economy.

In summary, critical examination of the report form used in automated electrocardiography showed a need for radical revision, insofar as the clinician was concerned. Such revision improved acceptance and cut costs both in time and in money. As a by-product, an entirely new method was made possible. This method enlisted cardiographers who were remote both from the processing centers and the hospitals served. As the speed of facsimile transmission improves, a flexible and economic system will result.

The Printout as the End Product of AMHT

H. A. Haessler, T. K. Holland and E. L. Elshtain

The print-out, the end product of the automated multiphasic health testing (AMHT) process, may be the basis upon which a doctor decides whether or not the testing procedure is useful. The preparation of any page of printed text involves several decisions concerning the available tools for producing the test. Some initial problems include selection of a typewriter, a type font and the general layout of a page. We have been considering the problem of formatting the contents of the print-out and have experimented with several designs. The following discussion will present those aspects we have found to be most important in presenting a readable and comprehensible print-out to the physician.

The first thing a doctor should want to know is what the patient's chief complaints are; why he has come to the office. Our self-administered questionnaire establishes this priority by means of a "rater" question. This question asks the patient to rate the importance of a preceding problem. Top priority problems appear at the very beginning of the print-out under the headings of "Primary Problems" and "Important Problems." Items of lesser importance follow these under the title "Symptomatic Review, Positive Responses." This section provides the physician with a broader view of the total health and habits of the patient. Subheadings report such general items as coffee drinking, smoking, use of alcohol or drugs and environmental exposure, as well as symptomatic organ systems.

Following the Symptomatic Review, the symptom groups which the patient has denied are listed. It was necessary to decide whether this negative data should list each individual symptom denied by the patient or be grouped by systems. The listing of particular items is so massive and forms such a formidable block of text that we chose to state only the organ systems or subsystems which are asymptomatic. This keeps the negative data to a minimum but still tells the doctor that all appropriate areas have been covered by the questionnaire.

Past illnesses are listed next and, finally, the various social, educational, employment, activity and familial history information. Thus the

H. A. Haessler, M.D., T. K. Holland *and* E. L. Elshtain, *Searle Medidata, Inc., Lexington, Mass.*

physician finds six major sections easily identifiable. This identification is aided through the use of headings at the left-most margin of the page. These headings are made even more apparent when two-case print is available.

The contents of each major section had to follow a logical order. This order serves a dual purpose: the physician must easily identify with the logic, as well as find it simple to follow. Therefore, we decided to use the usual pattern of any physical examination by proceeding from head to toe. This sequence is adhered to throughout the report.

With some information, most notably the social data, we have found a columnar format to be most efficacious, providing a sparse, highly readable and quickly noted organization of data.

The formatting of the physiological findings of the testing process also uses full capitalization for the major data divisions, such as ANTHRO-POMETRY, HEARING, VISION, BLOOD CHEMISTRY, etc. Within each section we have utilized either a basically vertical or a basically horizontal format. For example, hearing data follow a horizontal pattern, putting all threshold values in a line across from the appropriate ear. Blood chemistry data are put into a vertical or tabular format which allows the physician to scan down the list quickly for any particular test. The decision to use one basic organization rather than the other depends upon the type of data involved and how it may be most easily identified and comprehended, as well as how economically it can be printed.

Two other basic features needed to be explored: the visual separation of one block of data from another and emphasis for abnormal findings. We solved the former by the use of dotted lines. After each major division a line of dashes is typed across the page, clearly separating the end of one block from the beginning of the next. Abnormal data are flagged by typing asterisks adjacent to such information.

Another formatting problem was the provision of a chart of normal values for laboratory tests. We experimented briefly with a semigraphic format, but this resulted in a fairly formidable block of printed information. We have now included a parenthetic statement of the normal range whenever appropriate. This, plus the asterisks associated with abnormal values, allows the doctor to evaluate the magnitude of a particular finding.

This discussion has by no means exhausted all the possibilities for formatting the print-out of screening data. Consideration must be given to the content of each sentence of history information so that each begins with the symptom being discussed. Through further evolution, formats will continue to become more readable and easier to follow, with crucial data becoming more and more visible.

The Pre-Printed Form

Emerson Day

The report design which uses a pre-printed form and some of its advantages and disadvantages have been discussed. I would like to discuss these in more detail, using the pre-printed forms developed at Medequip as an example (Figs. 1-3).

The objective of the pre-printed format is to achieve maximum ease of reading for the fastest possible communication of data. Once the physician is familiar with the form, a quick glance over Page One (Fig. 1) will pick up the salient information regarding patient identification, socioeconomic and family background, habits, environment and past medical history. The contrast of blue pre-printing and black input typing increases scanability.

Page Two (Fig. 2) is open-ended for print-out of the review of systems by standard categories, using programmed crisp sentence structure based on the patient's responses to a branching history.

Page Three (Fig. 3) reverts to the pre-printed format for recording physiologic data and results of laboratory tests. It ends with an open section for the responsible physician's summary and recommendations with regard to further diagnostic procedures, therapy and management.

The family history section of Page One (Fig. 1) demonstrates a special example of design for rapid communication of information. By the use of X's in boxes, a clustering in vertical columns is telegraphed visually when a disease has been reported in multiple relatives. In this sample patient (disguised), a familial incidence of heart disease, hypertension and arthritis is highlighted and may be helpful to the physician responsible for her care. Other examples have been seen for tuberculosis and cancer. In one patient, a clustering of X's in the boxes under colitis for mother and for male and female relatives was the first clue to what proved to be familial polyposis.

Grouping of X's horizontally may also flag information of special significance, as in the profile of a patient reporting his father's death of stroke in the late forties together with a history of heart disease and hypertension.

Emerson Day, M.D., *Vice President and Director, Medequip Corporation, Park Ridge, Ill.*

159

Figure 1.

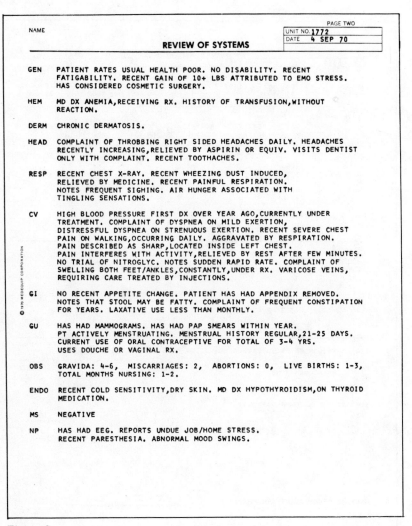

Figure 2.

When the family history is available and presented in this fashion, it can give the physician important information for the assessment and management of a patient being seen for the first time.

Similarly, the presentation of data concerning the patient's past history and habits in pre-established format, with which the physician quickly becomes familiar, delivers maximum information in minimum reading time.

PAGE THREE

UNIT NO.	1772
DATE	4 SEP 70
TIME	15:15

NAME

PHYSIOLOGICAL MEASUREMENTS

HEIGHT **67.9** INS WEIGHT **226** LBS SKIN FOLD **32** mm TEMP **97.3** F

CARDIOVASCULAR

			BLOOD PRESSURE
HEART RATE	84	/MIN	139/97
PULSE	85	/MIN	
PULSE DEFICIT			

PULMONARY

RESPIRATORY RATE	11	/MIN		
VITAL CAPACITY	2.5	L =	70	% NORM
FORCED EXPIR VOL – 1 SEC	2.07	L =	83	% OF VC
PEAK EXPIRATORY FLOW	4.11	L/SEC		

VISION ACUITY RELATIVE TO 20/30

	R EYE	L EYE	BOTH		
FAR	POORER	BETTER	BETTER	COLOR	NORMAL
NEAR	BETTER	BETTER	BETTER	PHORIA	NORMAL
TONOMETRY	22 mmHg	28 mmHg		DEPTH	NORMAL

HEARING THRESHOLD (db)

Hz	500	1000	2000	3000	4000	6000
RIGHT	36	28	16	18	19	23
LEFT	54	26	24	39	38	23

LABORATORY

HEMATOLOGY

HEMOGLOBIN	11.6	gm%
HEMATOCRIT	35.	%
RBC	4.1	$X10^6/mm^3$
MCV	85.	cu microns
MCH	28.	μμ gms
MCHC	33.	%
WBC	9900.	cu mm

SEROLOGY
NEG

BLOOD TYPE
O+

FECES
OCCULT BLOOD NEG

URINALYSIS

pH	5
PROTEIN	0
GLUCOSE	0
KETONES	0
OCCULT BLOOD	0

BLOOD CHEMISTRY

GLUCOSE	88.	mgm%	ALK PHOS	50.	mU/ml
GLUCOSE p̄ CHO	116.	mgm%	LDH	150.	mU/ml
URIC ACID	5.6	mgm%	SGOT	32.	mU/ml
BUN	14.	mgm%	TOTAL BILIRUBIN	0.8	mgm%
CHOLESTEROL	248.	mgm%	ALBUMIN	4.4	gm%
TRIGLYCERIDES	90.	mgm%	TOTAL PROTEIN	6.8	gm%
CALCIUM	9.6	mgm%	PBI	6.0	mcg%
PHOSPHORUS	3.3	mgm%			

ECG PROLONGED PR INTERVAL INDICATING FIRST DEGREE HEART BLOCK.

X-RAY CHEST - NSA
MAMMOGRAM - NSA

PAP TEST CLASS I,NEGATIVE.

SUMMARY AND RECOMMENDATIONS:

NSA= NO SIGNIFICANT ABNORMALITY ____________________ M.D.

Figure 3.

In our experience, the limitations which pre-printing places on ability to change the report form are more than offset by the advantages to the physician receiving the Patient Profile. In subsequent editions, more use is being made of X's in boxes (drugs, allergies and diet, for example). This further reduces print-out time and leaves adjacent space for annotations by the physician when he develops amplified information during his interview and examination.

Well-Patient Examinations:
Accessibility and Load on Facilities

Lawrence I. Schneider

For a variety of reasons, there is a shortage of physicians. This, of course, is nothing new and everyone knows that the net result is, and will continue to be, longer waits and higher fees for well patients wishing periodic examinations. Sick patients, too, will find it harder to obtain the services of a doctor who will accept them.

The answer to this manpower problem, at least in part, lies in better utilization of the physician's time. This is the premise for automated multiphasic health testing. Advocates of this approach, and I am one of them, say that the health care delivery system cannot afford for the physician to perform time-consuming routine tasks which render his time inefficient and ineffective. These fact-finding duties can be performed by the automated multiphasic health testing facility. Well-trained allied health personnel can efficiently and economically perform the necessary tasks to obtain reliable information, leaving the physician free to make the medical diagnosis.

The problem is in its implementation. The most common implementation has been in a linear layout where the examinee goes from station to station. Let's look at this type of facility from the standpoint of "accessibility" and "load on facilities."

The large, linear test facility is by nature centralized. People have to come to it, and they may have to come quite a distance for the most part. It is not accessible to the individual's own neighborhood. Testing in such a facility takes at least several hours; so it also may not be accessible from the point of view of time.

Looking at the load on such a facility, we find it not very flexible. It requires a large staff of testing personnel. If the load is not at its high programmed level, then the operation is costly and inefficient.

The linear layout has its place, but it also has drawbacks. A different approach is needed if testing is to be done on a decentralized level: in the

---

Lawrence I. Schneider, M.D., *President, International Health Systems, Inc., Rolling Meadows, Ill.*

163

neighborhood, in the plant or at other local sites. One facility that has worked successfully in filling this need is the single-station concept where most of the testing is done from one transportable testing console.

In the Computa-Lab system, the entire testing operation requires only 200 to 400 square feet of space and is performed by one to three testing technicians. As many as 50 persons a day can be tested, but the testing unit can operate economically and efficiently with a fraction of this patient load. Accessibility means having the test facility close, in distance and in time, to those individuals who need examinations.

The modular approach to automated multiphasic health testing is the desirable approach since it permits a representative complement of physiological testing devices to be compacted into a relatively small, easily transported configuration. This approach eliminates the undesirable features of a linear-type fixed facility by eliminating inflexibility and immobility.

Because of the lack of completely integrated, compact, mobile physiological testing stations, medicine is practiced today – out of necessity in many instances – on a symptomatic, i.e., "crisis," basis. As has been pointed out by many individuals in the past, this type of "symptomatic" medicine has been one of the great contributors to chronic disability and overcrowding of existing medical facilities. In addition, this approach has continued, not only because of the inability to administer the necessary "paramedical" tests prior to the patient's being seen by a physician, but also by the shortage of physicians to actually examine the patient and correlate physical findings with the profiling data available from the testing.

The approach of symptomatic or crisis medicine rather than preventive medicine has been reversed through the use of automated multiphasic health testing by a clinic in the Chicago area that is involved in publicly funded medical care of one type or another.

The Argyle Clinic, located in the uptown area of Chicago, had practiced purely symptomatic medicine in which a very limited amount of time could be devoted to each patient. The physicians involved in the operation of this clinic were well aware of the fact that they were not detecting predisposing conditions that would later lead to the development of a chronic disease state that could cause a patient to require additional, prolonged care and could even result in chronic disabling diseases, requiring long-term hospitalization and possible institutionalization in the future.

Again, the clinic was hampered in practicing preventive medicine by not being able to develop a good data base and profile on their patients. The patients going through the clinic did not receive any type of actual physical examination or paramedical testing that could be used to establish some type of a base for the patient. The development of such a program in this clinic, out of necessity, required a system that could be operated in a very limited physical area, would provide adequate testing and profiling by present standards, would generate the necessary hard copy of the patient's record and would also store these records in some type of a computer system so as to eliminate the "horrendous" paper empire generally associated with medical recordkeeping prior to the advent of the computer. Another important aspect was the ability to handle people, particularly in the history-taking area, who did not understand, read or speak English fluently without utilizing valuable personnel to administer history.

To this end, an audio approach to automated history taking is invaluable. In this particular instance, another consideration was the ability to move this equipment from the clinic into a temporary "store front" satellite-type of operation in order to bring the medical care closer to the people and, particularly, not to overload the existing fixed-clinic facility.

Utilizing a compact mobile approach as exemplified by the Computa-Lab System, the approach to their practice of medicine was changed from that of "crisis" to "preventive." The patients coming to the clinic with a specific complaint, such as a sore throat or pain in the abdomen, came for their appointment half an hour prior to the time they were scheduled to actually see the physician. They were put through the multiphasic system including all the usual parameters; at the time of the examination by the doctor, all the data, with the exception of laboratory, was immediately available. The physician, in addition to examining the patient relative to a specific complaint, was able to do an actual hands-on examination during the normal 15-30 minutes allocated to each patient. In most instances, this was the first time these people had been rendered a complete physical examination and evaluation of results in their entire life.

In reviewing the program as conducted at the Argyle Clinic from a medical and public health standpoint, it was apparent that the patient was now receiving medical care that had never been available to him before. Many conditions were detected in early stages that permitted evaluation and treatment so that, in terms of the future, the well-being of the individual patient, the eventual savings of public funds and, particularly, elimination of future over-crowding of public hospital facilities by these patients, actually became apparent. The physician now felt he was contributing total health care and offering much more benefit to the patient and community.

In summation, I have presented an actual instance of the use of a specific approach to automated multiphasic health testing to convert a private medical practice that served almost exclusively "welfare" patients in a symptomatic or crisis-type practice to one where these patients could be given physical examinations at regularly scheduled intervals, as had been advocated for many years by physicians but had been available only to their more affluent and economically sound fellow humans.

Major Problems in the Early Detection of Mental Illness

Roger Peele

The goal of detecting mental illness at an early stage, prior to its reaching a level of considerable discomfort or destruction, goes without question. Some of the ways that might initially come to mind in order to implement early detection are questionable, however.

In medicine, the well-patient examination is one of the most common ways of trying to achieve early detection, but psychiatry is not ready for such examinations. There are four reasons:

1. "Mentally well" has no agreed-upon definition. Sometimes we can answer a specific question of "Well enough to drive?", "Well enough to work?", but we could not answer the general question, "Is this person well?"

2. Rather than ask if the person is well, one might ask if the person shows early signs of "mental illness." But "mental illness" cannot be defined in precise, quantifiable characteristics either.

3. Even though the terms "mentally well" and "mental illness" offer no leads as to the possible usefulness of well-patient examinations, one might ask whether there are not criteria that would warn of impending mental illness. For nearly all mental illness categories, there is no concensus on cause and on only a few are there agreements on temporal antecedents. In some organic brain syndromes, there would be agreed-upon antecedents such as paresis. These detections need not be taken out of the regular medical examination.

4. A fourth problem around the well-patient examination in psychiatry is that our specialty includes clients other than the patient and includes others in the patient's environment, such as relatives, neighbors and employers. In the case of a very dangerous patient, for example, the needs of other clients take precedence over the wishes of the patient. In more subtle cases, it is frequently

Roger Peele, M.D., *Director, Area D Community Mental Health Center, Saint Elizabeth's Hospital, Washington, D. C.*

important to hear from these other people before one can decide whether there are problems to which one wants to apply the skills of mental health professionals. In psychiatry, examining only the well patient and not talking with those in his environment would be inadequate.

For these reasons, it is unlikely that the psychiatric well-patient examination is useful at the present time.

An allied approach to early detection may be the temptation to educate the public to make greater use of mental health services. This temptation may break the first rule of medicine: "to do no harm." It is quite difficult to carry out any public education that does not suggest that unhappiness, interpersonal difficulties or less than adequate functioning might be a result of mental illness and that mental health workers could assist with the complaints. This suggestion can be quite incorrect because of a lack of mental health workers and because of an actual inability of mental health workers to help with some problems. To the degree that people have problems which cannot be helped by mental health workers, we only add frustration to the problems with any suggestion they need help. There are enough "worried wells" already and we want to be careful not to expand the number even further.

Even if the well-patient examination and its associated public education are not valid approaches in psychiatry, early detection of mental illness can be increased by increasing the accessibility of mental health services. Accessibility can be increased by reducing financial barriers, waiting time, inconvenient appointment hours, logistic and travel barriers and the stigma of seeking mental health services.

There is always the fear that increased accessibility will lead to our services being overwhelmed. Without explaining in detail how to avoid being overwhelmed, we will only list some of the methods we have used. In presenting the following list, we do not mean to suggest that carrying out these suggestions is without problems:

1. Generalize the roles of the staff in the mental health organization.
2. Keep the clinical decisions at the so-called lowest level in the organization.
3. Related to this, decentralize responsibility for clinical decisions.
4. Develop comprehensive services.
5. Develop these comprehensive services in one location.
6. Use the least expensive personnel when other factors are equal.
7. Develop the role of the most expensive individual of the organization so that he can have the broadest impact.
8. Avoid any rigid delineation of the term "mental illness."
9. Increase the awareness of the staff concerning costs.

Summary

In psychiatry, there are some major obstacles to the implementation of one of the major tools in the early detection of illness — the well-patient examination. These obstacles include a lack of definition of "mentally well" or "mentally ill" and a lack of concensus on the causes of mental illness. Another obstacle is the fact that in psychiatry one is often serving, besides the patient himself, persons in the patient's environment. This paper not only summarizes the difficulties but also explains why some efforts to overcome these difficulties may have an adverse effect and increase the number of "worried well."

Even though the well-patient examination is not a tool for detection of early mental illness, increasing the accessibility of early mental health services in general certainly increases early detection. Increased accessibility leads to fears of overwhelming the services. This paper reviews some of the ways of avoiding being overwhelmed.

Value of Biochemical Profiling in a Periodic Health Examination Program: Analysis of 1000 Cases

W. R. Cunnick, J. B. Cromie, Ruth Cortell, Barbara Wright,
Eliot Beach, Frederic Seltzer and Sybil Miller

Introduction

The rediscovery of health screening in the last few years has led to broad expectations about its future. Addition of automated technology and computer techniques have provided a new tool, the Multiphasic Health Screening System. It is hoped that this system can help establish priorities for medical treatment, extend health care to those not receiving it, establish diagnoses at earlier stages of disease and possibly retard spiraling health care costs.

As we proceed to experiment with new health maintenance systems, it is appropriate to periodically review what we are doing and try to make value judgments. In this paper we will do so in regard to one component of these new systems, Biochemical Profiling. Two kinds of evidence will be presented:

1. A statistical analysis of the results of Biochemical Profiling in 1000 consecutive periodic health exams, to which this form of testing was added for the first time.
2. Observations and case reports based on our three years' experience with approximately 15,000 profiles done at periodic examinations.

Background and Methods

The Metropolitan Life Insurance Company purchased an SMA 12/30 AutoAnalyzer in March 1967, with three objectives in mind:

1. To determine whether this new information would facilitate early diagnosis, treatment and prevention of employee illness.

W. R. Cunnick, M.D., J. B. Cromie, M.D., Ruth Cortell, M.D., Barbara Wright, M.D., Eliot Beach, Ph.D., Frederic Seltzer, FSA, and Sybil Miller, *Metropolitan Life Insurance Company, New York, N. Y. The senior author is Medical Director.*

2. To evaluate the possible role of biochemical profiles in life insurance underwriting.

3. To gain experience in the emerging field of bioengineering technology.

Our first step was to establish the range of normal values for healthy persons (Table 1). This was done by testing employees of different sex and age ranges who were known to be in good health. No hemolyzed or otherwise imperfect sera were submitted to the AutoAnalyzer. Bio-chemical values were charted on an optical scan sheet and punch cards produced by an IBM 1232 Optical Scan Reader. Distribution of normal values was ascertained using a 95% confidence interval.[1]

The present study concerns itself with an analysis of 1000 approximately consecutive biochemical profiles done on Home Office employees (New York City) over age 35. These were performed early in 1968 as part of the periodic health examination. It is important to recognize that extensive health records already existed on these persons, including diagnostic coding, sporadic biochemistry results, etc. The charts were studied two years later and the following classification of results was developed:

A. Positives

　　1. New Positive Case: Employee record with abnormal biochemical value(s) leading to diagnosis of a previously unknown disease entity or pathophysiological biochemical syndrome.

　　2. Confirmatory Positive Case: Employee record with abnormal biochemical value(s) confirming previously known disease or syndrome.

　　3. Unclassified Positive Case: Employee record with abnormal bio-chemical value(s) of no apparent diagnostic significance. We prefer the term "unclassified" to "false" positive; the latter term implies that misleading information has been provided. Most "unclassified" positives are, in fact, only the result of statistical formulations of the "normal" range, which defines cases falling in the upper and lower 2.5% of values as "abnormal." These ranges are chosen to avoid an excessive number of referrals for further evaluation.[1]

B. Negatives

　　　Employee records with all 12 biochemical values within the normal ranges according to age and sex. We recognize that there may be "false" negative values among this group, but no detailed search was made for them as this investigation was concerned primarily with the "positive" group.

Statistical Results

In the evaluation of multiphasic health screening systems, one of the central questions is what are we trying to find? Historically, our concepts of a "disease" entity have rested on combinations of information about etiology, pathology, course of illness, response to treatment and prognosis. However, as medicine moves into more intricate biochemistry, and beyond that into molecular pathophysiology and genetics, the concept of "disease" must be expanded. For these reasons we have classified our New Positive Cases into either recognized disease entities or pathophysiological biochemical syndromes (Table 2). For example, it is probably more important for a person to know he has a hypercholesterolemic "syndrome," which may be altered, than Paget's disease, which requires no treatment.

It is probably not unexpected that Table 2 reveals diabetes mellitus as the most frequent newly discovered disease. Biochemical profiling has also been useful in finding unsuspected alcoholic liver disease (See Case Reports and Observations). Deviations in calcium and phosphorus suggestive of hyperparathyroidism are discovered in routine profiling: whether these findings alone justify exploration for parathyroid adenoma is a matter of debate.[2]

In Group A (Table 2), the case of cholelithiasis was found following investigation of an elevated serum bilirubin. The case of "drug hepatitis" occurred in a person taking theophylline diuretics for many years: abnormal liver enzymes reverted to normal ranges after cessation of the drug.

In Group B (Table 2), the hypercholesterolemic syndromes were most frequent. Their significance as a coronary risk factor is well known. A simple method for further classification of hyperlipidemic states is described in the section on Case Reports and Observations.

Also in Group B (Table 2), cases of secondary hyperuricemia were all related to thiazide therapy. There is some indication that any diuretic which contracts extracellular fluid volume will raise serum uric acid levels,[3] and secondary acute gout is occasionally seen.

Turning to the Confirmatory Positive Cases (Table 3), in which no new diagnoses were made, a preponderance of diabetes mellitus is seen. The case of congestive heart failure was associated with elevated serum LDH levels, as were those of lymphosarcoma and myeloid metaplasia. We are convinced that clinicians should not be too casual in dismissing isolated elevated LDH values. While it is known that they can be associated with a wide variety of conditions in symptomatic persons,[4] our experience suggests that it can be an early indicator of a developing myeloproliferative

TABLE 1. Biochemical Profiles in a Healthy Employee Population
Distribution of Values – Classified by Age and Sex*

Observed Values†		Chol. (mg%)	CA (mg%)	Biochemical Profile (SMA 12) In. Phos. (mg%)	T. Bil. (mg%)	Alb. (gm%)	T. Prot. (gm%)
Males							
Under Age 35	(L)	147.6	9.4	2.5	0.2	3.8	6.7
	(H)	283.4	10.8	4.3	1.2	5.0	8.3
Ages 35-44	(L)	158.3	9.0	2.3	0.0	3.6	6.5
	(H)	320.3	11.0	4.3	1.6	5.0	8.3
Ages 45-54	(L)	174.3	9.0	2.3	0.2	3.5	6.5
	(H)	323.9	10.8	4.1	1.2	4.9	8.3
Ages 55 and Over	(L)	172.6	9.1	2.1	0.2	3.5	6.4
	(H)	313.8	10.7	4.1	1.2	4.7	8.2
Technicon Normal Ranges	(L)	150.0	8.5	2.5	0.2	3.5	6.0
	(H)	300.0	10.5	4.5	1.0	5.0	8.0
Females							
Under Age 35	(L)	138.3	9.2	2.5	0.2	3.6	6.5
	(H)	270.9	10.6	4.3	1.0	4.8	8.3
Ages 35-44	(L)	152.9	9.1	2.4	0.2	3.5	6.5
	(H)	299.7	10.7	4.4	1.0	4.7	8.3
Ages 45-54	(L)	168.4	9.0	2.5	0.2	3.4	6.4
	(H)	342.6	10.8	4.5	1.0	4.6	8.2
Ages 55 and Over	(L)	189.1	9.1	2.7	0.3	3.3	6.5
	(H)	346.9	10.9	4.5	0.9	4.7	8.1

Observed Values†	Uric Ac. (mg%)	BUN (mg%)	Glucose (mg%)	LDH (W.U.)	Alk. Phos. (K.A.U.)	SGOT (W.U.)
Males						
Under Age 35	4.0	9.3	69.0	67.8	6.1	7.9
	8.8	22.1	106.8	120.6	14.9	41.9
Ages 35-44	3.8	8.6	69.9	72.0	4.2	1.3
	9.0	24.4	112.7	127.2	16.8	55.5
Ages 45-54	3.9	9.3	70.8	74.7	4.3	6.2
	8.9	24.7	121.0	132.9	18.3	48.6
Ages 55 and Over	3.9	9.2	64.8	74.7	4.2	10.8
	9.1	26.4	129.8	129.7	18.2	41.6
Technicon Normal Ranges	2.5	10.0	65.0	30.0	4.0	10.0
	8.0	20.0	110.0	120.0	17.0	40.0
Females						
Under Age 35	2.7	7.4	62.4	62.2	4.8	10.9
	6.1	19.2	95.2	114.2	12.6	28.3
Ages 35-44	2.5	6.1	62.7	77.2	3.2	10.9
	6.7	22.9	117.1	121.4	16.0	33.9
Ages 45-54	2.7	8.8	64.1	72.3	4.0	5.7
	7.1	24.2	119.9	137.1	17.6	42.5
Ages 55 and Over	2.8	9.3	61.4	81.2	4.6	7.0
	7.8	26.1	126.4	136.8	19.0	43.6

(L) Low
(H) High
* Presented at the Technicon International Symposium, Chicago, Illinois, June 5, 1969.
† 95% interval

TABLE 2. Results

New Positives
A. Recognized Disease Entity inferring well-known features of
   etiology, pathology and prognosis.

Diabetes mellitus	3
Alcoholic liver disease	2
Paget's disease	2
Hyperparathyroidism	2
Cholelithiasis	1
Drug hepatitis	1
	11

B. Pathophysiological Biochemical Syndromes having recognized
   features of etiology and prognosis, in which many physicians
   would advise further investigation and/or treatment.

Primary hypercholesterolemia	7
Hyperuricemia secondary to hypertensive therapy	5
Constitutional hyperbilirubinemia	1
Total	24 (2.4%)

TABLE 3. Results

Confirmatory Positives

Diabetes mellitus	20
Primary hypercholesterolemia	4
Secondary hypercholesterolemia (hypothyroid)	2
Gout	4
Alcoholic liver disease	2
Cholelithiasis	1
Congestive heart failure	1
Hypoparathyroidism	1
Benign prostatic hypertrophy	1
Lymphosarcoma	1
Myeloid metaplasia	1
Total	38 (3.8%)

disorder in nonsymptomatic cases. Physicians may wish to keep these
patients under review for hematologic study at appropriate intervals.

The Unclassified Positive Cases are illustrated in Table 4. There were
225 unclassified abnormal values occurring in 190 cases. These cases result
largely from the definition of the "normal range," as discussed above. The
bell-shaped Gaussian distribution curve has its limitations when used to
describe some biological systems. For instance, in physiological terms
there may be no such thing as a "high serum albumin" or "low LDH."
Many of the "high albumins" in the Unclassified Positive Group were
probably related to slight degrees of hemolysis.

TABLE 4. Unclassified Positive Values in 190 Cases

Test	No. High	No. Low	Total
1. Cholesterol	0	14	14
2. Calcium	10	0	10
3. Inorg. phosphatase	12	17	29
4. T. bilirubin	17	0	17
5. Albumin	50	1	51
6. T. protein	8	2	10
7. Uric acid	9	8	17
8. BUN	12	1	13
9. Glucose	4	7	11
10. LDH	7	26	33
11. Alk. phosphatase	11	0	11
12. SGOT	9	0	9
Total			225

A summary of our experience is seen in Table 5, where it can be observed that the yield of new information considered to be significant was 2.4%; Confirmatory Positives, 3.8%; Unclassified Positives, 19.0%; and Negatives, 74.8%. Many workers in the multiphasic health screening field believe any component must have a new yield between 0.5% and 2.0% to justify inclusion in the system, in order not to produce an excessive number of referrals for further evaluation. It is our opinion that biochemical profiling meets these criteria for inclusion.

Case Reports and Observations

After three years' experience with approximately 15,000 biochemical profiles done with periodic health examinations, the following observations are offered:

1. *Routine biochemical profiling aids* in the detection and management of alcoholism in the Occupational Health Maintenance System. This is especially true in women, many of whom have great difficulty recognizing that they have a drinking problem. The

TABLE 5. Summary

	No. of Cases	%
A. Positives		
1. New Positives	24	2.4
a. Recognized disease entity	11	1.1
b. Pathophysiological biochemical syndrome	13	1.3
2. Confirmatory Positives	38	3.8
3. Unclassified Positives	190	19.0
B. Negatives	748	74.8
Total	1000	100.0

profile sheet itself serves as a visual aid and is often highly useful in convincing an employee that objective evidence indicates a problem. If possible, the diagnosis of alcoholism must also be substantiated by means other than the biochemical profile alone. Otherwise, it remains a "probable" diagnosis.

Early alcoholic liver disease shows moderate elevations of SGOT and LDH. Later there are rises in alkaline phosphatase and bilirubin. When the cirrhotic stage is reached, the albumin and BUN may fall, with rises in total protein due to hyperglobulinemia.

Cessation of drinking and participation in a rehabilitation program are correlated with return of the biochemical profile toward normal, depending on the stage of the disease.

An illustrative case (Figs. 1-4) is that of an employee who was seen for periodic medical examination in July 1969. There were no symptoms, history or physical findings to suggest a health problem. Routine biochemical profile, however, showed substantial elevations of SGOT and LDH (Fig. 1). (Uric acid was also high and he has subsequently had clinical gout.) Five months later, in response to reduced alcohol intake, the profile showed lower levels of LDH and SGOT (Fig. 2). Possibly encouraged by improvement in the profile, he resumed alcohol consumption, and a routine profile in July 1970 showed increased levels of LDH and SGOT (Fig. 3). Concerned about continued abnormality of the biochemical profile, he stopped all alcohol consumption. Three months later the profile was normal (Fig. 4).

2. *Cases are occasionally seen* in which the abnormal biochemical profile gives the only indication of deterioration in the health status of the employee:

Mr. C. was a 61-year-old man who for a number of years had heavy albuminuria and slight elevation of BUN (Fig. 5). He continued to work and had no symptoms. In April 1970, a routine biochemical profile showed significant change; with rise in BUN, fall in serum albumin and a rising phosphorus (Fig. 6). Alerted by this unexpected change, he was seen at more frequent intervals. Five months later a repeat profile showed alarming deterioration, with further rise in BUN and phosphorus and with falling albumin and calcium (Fig. 7). In cooperation with his personal physician, he was referred to a kidney failure treatment center where dialysis and transplant were available if necessary.

In this case, routine profiling prevented this kidney failure from reaching an advanced stage unrecognized; dialysis could be done as an elective rather than emergency procedure. It is possible that a death was prevented or delayed.

Mr. Z. was a 60-year-old man who said he felt well, although indirect reports suggested he was functioning poorly. Physical examination was negative. The biochemical profile (Fig. 8) showed several highly abnormal results: glucose over 500, elevated alkaline

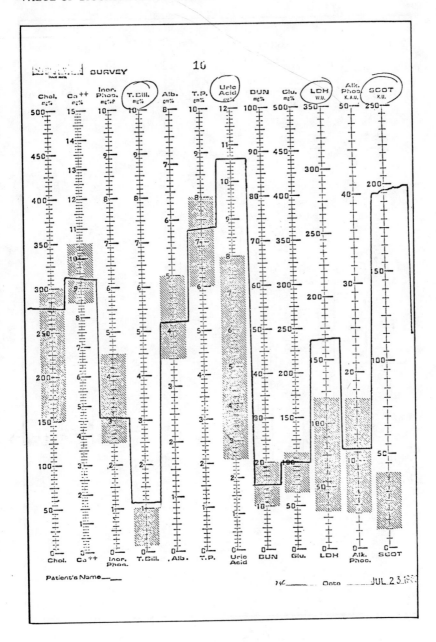

Figure 1.

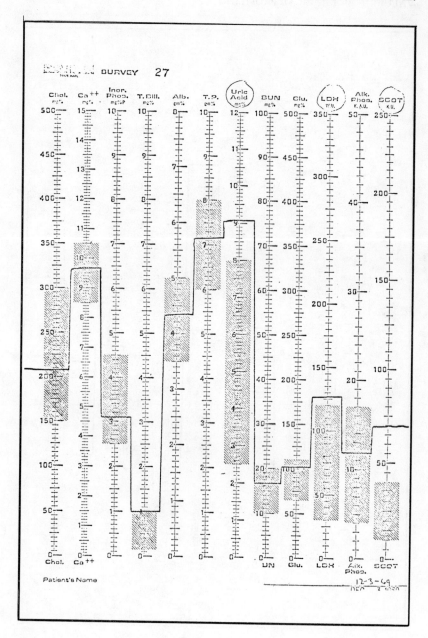

Figure 2.

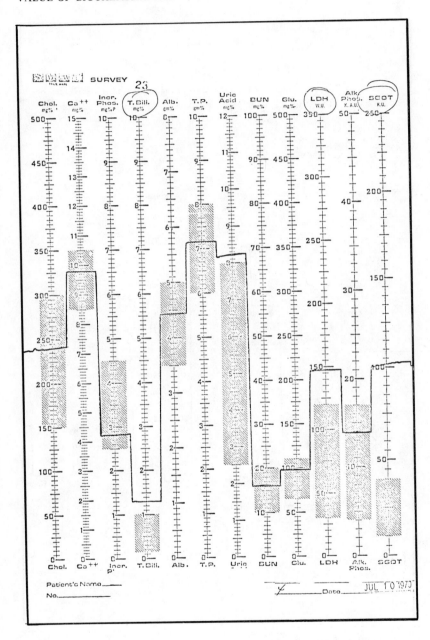

Figure 3.

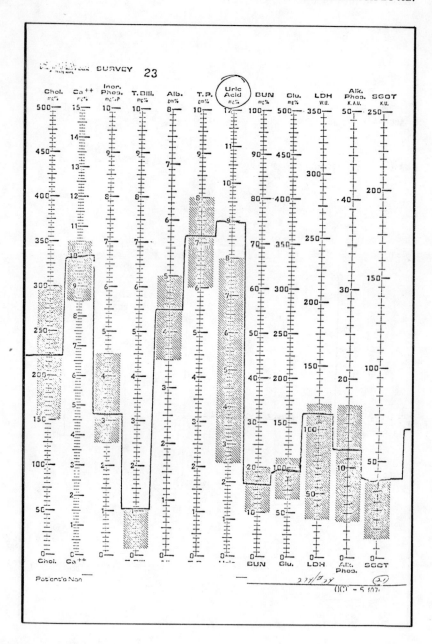

Figure 4.

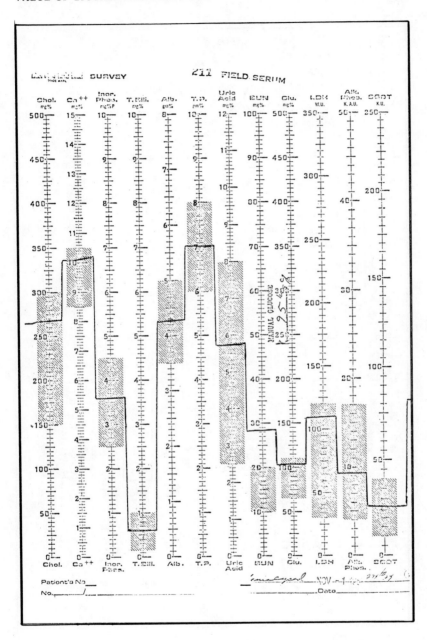

Figure 5.

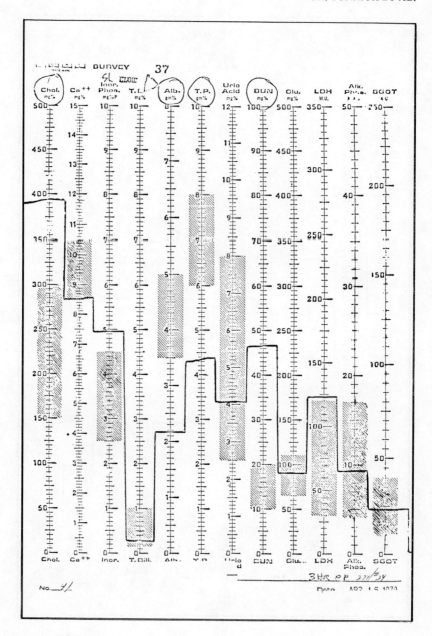

Figure 6.

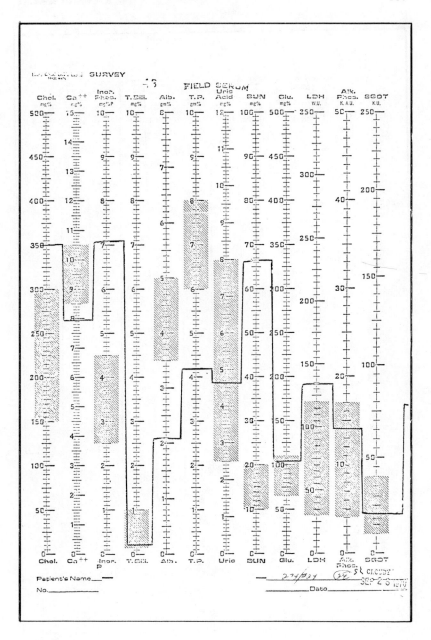

Figure 7.

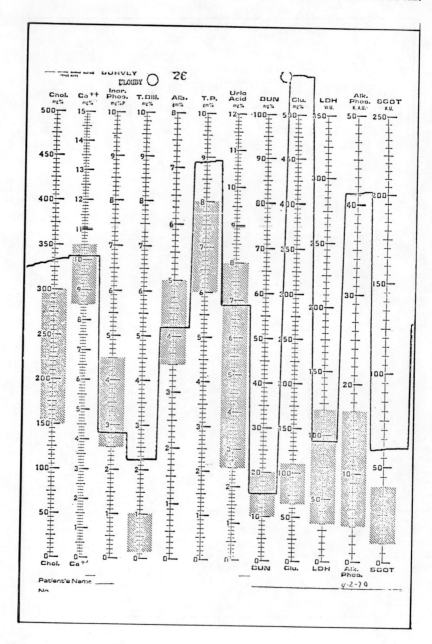

Figure 8.

phosphatase and bilirubin. An immediate investigation was begun by his personal physician, but he died suddenly ten days later. No autopsy was performed, but a diagnosis of carcinoma of the pancreas could explain the biochemical abnormalities and sudden death by thrombosis or embolism. This case is notable in that the only evidence of the seriousness of his condition came from the biochemical profile.

3. *Use of routine biochemical profiling detects* persons with elevated cholesterol levels, a known coronary risk factor, which can be reduced by appropriate diet and drugs.

A screening classification of the most common hyperlipoproteinemic states can be done by relatively simple procedures as follows: All sera are allowed to stand overnight in a refrigerator, then compared against a set of standards for turbidity. A simple phenol turbidity test is also done. Neutral glycerides are determined if either of these tests is abnormal. In this way a screening classification can be made (Fig. 9), which is adequate for clinical purposes.

Summary

Addition of biochemical profiling to a periodic health examination system among a group of active, employed persons *who already had extensive medical records* resulted in a 2.4% yield of new information considered to be significant.

It is reasonable to assume that if the biochemical profiling were done on a similar population without previous health records, the yield of new information would be approximately 4%-6%. Likewise, if the profiling is repeated subsequently on the same population, the yield would probably be in the range of 1%.

The most frequent conditions newly encountered were hypercholesterolemic and hyperuricemic states, diabetes mellitus and alcoholic liver

Type of Hyperlipoproteinemia[5]	Cholesterol	Neutral Glycerides	Recommendation
II	↑	Usually Normal or Decreased	Weight control, low cholesterol diet, emphasis on polyunsaturated fats
IV	N or ↓	Usually Increased	Weight control, relative restriction of carbohydrates[5]

Fig. 9. Types II and IV account for the largest number of cases in the Fredrickson Classification.[5] At the present time we are not using lipoprotein electrophoresis, but we may use it for selected cases in the future.

disorders. A screening system has been developed for further classification of the hyperlipidemic states.

Experience with biochemical profiling in the occupational health setting has shown it useful in detecting and rehabilitating alcoholic cases.

Persons are occasionally seen in whom an abnormal or changing biochemical profile gives the only clue to serious or progressive illness.

References

1. Cunnick, W. R., Cromie, J. B., Beach, E. F. et al.: Biochemical profiles in a healthy employee population: Distribution of values classified by age and sex. *Advances in Automated Analysis* (Vol. 3, Technicon International Congress, 1969.) New York:Mediad Inc., 1970, pp. 85-88.
2. Ahlvin, R. C.: Biochemical screening − A critique. *New Eng. J. Med.,* 283:1084-1086, 1970.
3. Weilerstein, R.: Diuretics and hyperuricemia. *New Eng. J. Med.,* 283:1170, 1970.
4. Glick, J. H. Jr.: Serum lactate dehydrogenase isoenzyme and total lactate dehydrogenase values in health and disease, and clinical evaluation of these tests by means of discriminant analysis. *Amer. J. Clin. Path.,* 52:320-328, 1969.
5. Fredrickson, D. S., Levy, R. I. and Lees, R. S.: Fat transport in lipoproteins − An integrated approach to mechanisms and disorders. *New Eng. J. Med.,* 276:34-44, 94-103, 148-156, 215-225, 273-281, 1967.

This paper was published in the *Bulletin of the New York Academy of Medicine*, January 1972, and is reprinted by permission.

Automated Urinalysis: Feasibility and Clinical Value

DeWitt T. Hunter, Jr. and Philip A. Fidel

There are two basic approaches to clinical laboratory testing. These are quantitative analyses and qualitative estimations. In general, the cost and effort input of quantitative approaches are high. Qualitative, or "spot testing," has the advantage of low cost but sacrifices accuracy.[1] In recent years, the trend has been away from qualitative approaches. This is in part due to efforts to afford better health care delivery, but mainly due to extended analytic capability through automation.

Automation is being increasingly utilized in virtually all areas of the laboratory.[2] Direct benefits resulting from automation include enhanced accuracy and precision, decreased professional effort and significant decrease in cost to the patient.[3] Automation also provides rapid mass screening and maximum quality control capability. In addition, with computer interface, equipment can be monitored with further gains in time, quality control and economy. Data may be rapidly collated, retrieved and made available for vital diagnostic analysis.[4]

Urinalysis, the assay of urine constituents, is the last major area in which manual qualitative testing is still widely performed.[5] The routine urinalysis consists of a pH determination, a specific gravity measurement, an occult blood or hemoglobin screen, a carbohydrate test, a test for albumin and a microscopic examination of the sediment.[6] Urinalysis, one of the most common test batteries, is performed on every hospital admission, in doctors' offices and in all out-patient clinics. It is an integral component of every health examination performed. Many clinicians feel that the urinalysis is the single most important examination performed on a given patient. Insurance companies require that such an analysis accompany all physical examinations, and more often than not, this is the only laboratory study performed. Yet, with the exception of qualitative or crude semi-quantitative tests, few advances have been made within the last decade. Although automation has proceeded rapidly in all areas of the laboratory field, minimal progress has occurred in the field of urinalysis.

DeWitt T. Hunter, Jr., M.D. *and* Philip A. Fidel, M.S., *Latter-Day Saints Hospital, Salt Lake City, Utah.*

We undertook studies on the feasibility of enhancing the accuracy, precision and clinical value of conventional urinalysis. It was soon recognized that these aims could best be achieved through automation. Since existing automated apparatuses are primarily designed to analyze serum metabolites, it was soon found necessary to radically redesign existing systems to properly analyze urine. This was necessary because the chemical constituents and physical characteristics of urine differ greatly from serum. Challenging problems were repeatedly encountered, defined and, for the most part, solved. Promising new methodologies and components were devised.

Equipment

Continuous flow systems were assembled from basic Technicon (Technicon Instruments Inc., Tarrytown, N. Y.) and Beckman (Beckman Instruments Inc., Fullerton, Calif.) elements. Special manifolds were constructed and proportion pumps were used to deliver reagents and specimens. An AutoAnalyzer sampler was used to sequence and time specimen sampling. Dialysis was performed where needed using either a long or short SMA 12/60 dialyzer.

Optical density readings were obtained using a Beckman DB-G spectrophotometer with a 10-inch linear-log recorder. The recorder was set for log mode at 1 inch per minute. Fifteen millimeter (15 mm) quartz flow-through cells were used with the apparatus.

Test Systems

Chemical procedures and requisite flow systems were developed to assay urine bilirubin, creatinine, glucose, hemoglobin, ketone and protein. Specific gravity was estimated by conductivity.

A simple but very effective method was developed to analyze bilirubin, which absorbs maximally in the 440 nm range. The conjugated form is very labile and is readily oxidized with ablation of its maxima. Dilute hypochlorite was used to effect this oxidation. The difference in absorption at 440 was equated to bilirubin concentration.

$$\text{Bilirubin} \quad \xrightarrow{\text{Oxidizing Agent}} \quad \text{Urobilinogen}$$
$$440 \text{ nm} \qquad\qquad\qquad (\text{Colorless})$$

Creatinine was measured using the Jaffe[7] reaction, which yields a red color when reacted with picric acid in the presence of a strong alkali.

Creatinine + Alkaline Picrate → Red Tautomer of Creatinine

Glucose was assayed using a conjugated enzymatic sequence: hexokinase and ATP phosphorylate glucose to glucose-6-phosphate. Glucose-6-

phosphate dehydrogenase then oxidizes glucose-6-phosphate to gluconolactone-6-phosphate. The coenzymes NADP and TNADP (Thio-NADP) act as hydrogen acceptors and are reduced to NADPH and TNADPH. This reduction bears a direct molar ratio to glucose conversion. Absorbance of NADPH is read at 340 nm and TNADPH is read at 400 nm. The basic system using NADP only was described in detail by Peterson.[8] TNADP was used to facilitate visual reading and regulation of sensitivity.

$$\text{HK}$$
$$\text{Glucose + ATP} \rightarrow \text{G-6P + ADP}$$

$$\text{G-6-PDH}$$
$$\text{G-6P+NADP-TNADP} \quad \rightarrow \quad \text{Gluconolactone-6-phosphate+}$$
$$\text{(Colorless)} \qquad\qquad \text{NADPH-TNADPH}$$
$$\text{(Yellow)}$$

A highly sensitive method was developed to estimate hemoglobin concentration. Hemoglobin acts as a peroxidase to catalyze the oxidation of colorless oxygen acceptors to chromogenic states in the presence of hydrogen peroxide.

$$\text{Hgb (peroxidase)}$$
$$o\text{-Dianisidine} \quad \rightarrow \quad \text{Oxidized O-Dianisidine}$$
$$\text{(Colorless)} \qquad\qquad \text{(Red-Yellow)}$$

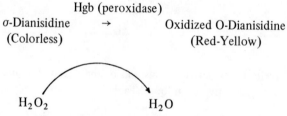

$$H_2O_2 \qquad\qquad H_2O$$

Sodium nitroferricyanide reacts with ketones in the presence of an alkali to form a lavender to deep-purple color.[9]

$$\text{Oxidized acetoacetic acid}$$
$$\text{Na Nitroprusside + Acetoacetic} \rightarrow \text{(Blue - Violet)}$$
$$\text{Acid}$$

Urine protein was estimated by the sulfosalicylic acid precipitation technique. The degree of turbidity is proportional to the quantity of proteins present.[10]

Population Study

Twenty normal people of both sexes were studied to establish normal limits for these studies. Approximately 100 randomly selected patients were studied. In addition to the automated procedures, each specimen was analyzed by one or more reference procedures. Glucose, ketones, protein, bile and hemoglobin were all presumptively tested using the Ames Bili-Lab-Stix. Creatinine was assayed by an automated method[7] and glucose was, in addition, estimated by a colorimetric procedure.[11] All specimens in which a discrepancy was encountered were assayed by an additional reference procedure. These confirmative procedures included the Acetest for ketones, the sulfosalycylic acid turbidimetric test for protein, the Ictotest for bile and the Hematest for hemoglobin.

Results

Table 1 summarizes the normal limits observed and the reproducibility of the various chemical tests.

TABLE 1. Normal Ranges and Reproducibility of Various Test Systems

Metabolite	Range mg/100 ml	Coefficient of Variance
Creatinine	20-340	3.6%
Glucose	0-14	7.6%
Hemoglobin	0-2	7.1%
Ketone	4-24	4.3%
Protein	0-0.6	8.6%
Bilirubin	0-0.2	8.0%

The quantitative sensitivity threshold of the automated approach was superior to the qualitative techniques. Table 2 shows this analysis.

TABLE 2. Comparative Threshold Detection

Test System	Quantitative mg/100 ml	Qualitative mg/100 ml	Observed Upper Limit of Normal mg/100 ml
Creatinine	350*	20*	340*
Glucose	5	10 (Kark)	26
Hemoglobin	2	2 (Kark)	2.057
Ketones	5	10 (Kark)	24
Total Protein	0.6	20 (Kark)	0.6
Bilirubin	0.02	0.05 (Kark)	0.03

*Creatinine is normally present in high concentration. Conventional methods use great dilution to enable scale reading. Values in the table are presented in terms of upper rather than lower threshold levels.

Creatinine concentration was studied from a standpoint of establishing its value as a reference in expressing metabolite excretion rate. This data is shown in Table 3.

TABLE 3. Normal Metabolite Ranges
24-Hour Excretion Values vs. Creatinine Concentration

Metabolite	Normal Range mg/24 Hr.	Normal Range mg/mg Creatinine × 1000
Glucose	0-153	0-86
Hemoglobin	0-35	0-27
Ketone	30-285	20-160
Protein	0-9	0-4
Bilirubin	0-0.5	0-0.3

Thirty-one patients were detected in whom one or more chemical values were abnormal. The results of these abnormal studies are shown in Table 4.

TABLE 4. Comparison of Elevated Metabolite Levels Encountered in Patients — Quantitative Tests vs. Qualitative Tests

Metabolite	No. Elevated by Quantitative Method	No. Elevated by Qualitative Method
Glucose	15	9
Hemoglobin	6	5
Ketone	8	1
Protein	17	12
Bilirubin	4	2

Discussion

Routine urinalysis, as presently performed in clinical laboratories throughout the country has afforded a means for rapid and economic mass screening of patients. Significant changes in metabolism secondary to diseases such as diabetes, kidney infection, hemolytic anemias, liver disease and a variety of pathologic processes that alter the "normal" composition of urine are usually detected. The semi-quantitative "spot tests" are simple to perform and require a minimum of experience or skill at interpreting color changes. However, the reputed sensitivity, specificity and quantitative accuracy of spot testing has been questioned.[5,12] As virtually all other areas of laboratory science advance, clinical microscopy has remained static and progressively its relative importance decreases.

Through automation, it was possible to analyze urine at a more rapid rate than it could be done manually, with greater sensitivity, accuracy and precision. Most significantly, the metabolites could be quantitated and even reported in terms of excretion rates. Under normal conditions the volume of urine excreted inversely relates to the concentration of urine metabolites. Using creatinine excretion as a reference point (the 24-hour excretion of creatinine is reasonably constant for individuals of the same sex), dilution and concentration effects can be eliminated. Few clinicians will argue that precise quantitation of urine metabolites, using test systems with extremely low detection thresholds, has considerable clinical justification. Low-threshold detection will enable incipient disease to be detected at an earlier stage, while precise quantitation will enable the diseases to be more closely scrutinized for therapeutic effects.

One of the most important considerations of automated systems over manual procedures is the decrease in overall cost. With the automation of urinalysis, a decrease in the total cost for a test should be realized despite the incorporation of additional tests. As with chemical screening, the unit cost per test decreases with the number of tests performed. In general, work patterns and specimen flow can be made more efficient. Statistical data can be gathered more efficiently and evaluated. Accordingly, there will also be a decrease in false-positive and false-negative results due to human error. Conservation of personnel effort will enable extension into new laboratory efforts. More time and study can be devoted to the microscopic examination of the urinary sediment.

Several innovations have been incorporated in the feasibility study. Threshold detection has been enhanced through the photometric readout (Table 4). Test systems have been modified or developed to meet certain mechanical restrictions or clinical requirements. One completely new modification involves the glucose test system.

The measurement of true glucose by any method has always met with formidable difficulties. Quantitation by the ATP-hexokinase method of Peterson[8] has been widely accepted; however, it has not been adapted to urine analysis. The great sensitivity of the test limited the effective range. In addition, readings were made in the ultraviolet range at 340 nm. By adding Thio-NADP to the reaction mixture, the test can be read in the visible 400 nm range. The NADP-TNADP ratio can be adjusted to permit a range excursion to over 1000 mg/100 ml without specimen dilution. It is virtually interference free. The capability to detect minute elevations of urine glucose may facilitate the detection of early diabetes.

Another new modification was the quantitation of bilirubin by direct oxidation with sodium hypochlorite. Normal values established for this method are comparable to the sensitivity required of spot tests. This test provides a sensitive means for quantitating and detecting incipient cases of hepatitis and other hepatic diseases.[13]

The presence of hemoglobin in urine has great significance in the detection of hemolytic disease, bleeding diathesis and numerous genito-urinary tract diseases. O-dianisidine was employed to provide greater sensitivity than benzidine, the commonly used chromogen. Dianisidine is approximately five times more sensitive to peroxidase activity than other benzidine derivatives.[14] Quantities as low as 3 mg/100 ml are detected. In this low range, hemoglobin is usually present as the result of shed red cells.

Ketone bodies are measured by means of a modified nitroprusside test. Ammonia hydroxide is added to prevent interference by creatinine. The test is sufficiently sensitive to detect low-grade metabolic acidosis due to starvation, malnutrition or poor glucose metabolism. Debilitated patients with complicating conditions cannot be adequately evaluated using qualitative tests.

Total protein is usually measured on random morning specimens. For maximum information, a 24-hour specimen is usually analyzed to establish increasing or decreasing pathologic trends. The use of sulfosalicylic acid as the precipitating agent will allow the detection of proteoses which are excreted during active, progressive renal disease. Furthermore, abnormal proteins, such as Bence-Jones protein fragments, are important in the diagnosis of blood dyscrasias. Serial urine examinations by quantitative protein tests in the third trimester of pregnancy may pick up early rises and enable the early diagnosis of eclampsia. Numerous other examples could be given.

Introduction of automation into urinalysis with digital reporting will require a certain amount of re-education. As quantitative data are accumulated for normal and pathologic states, the relationship between the various results must be related to the clinical picture. At a future time, the analysis and evaluation of urine metabolites will be of the same degree as that accorded serum findings.

Several additional tests may be adapted to automated urine analysis. These include methods for detecting phenylketonuria and other inborn errors of metabolism, as well as tests for chloride and other ions, urobilinogen, bacteria, various enzymes, toxological derivatives and medications.

Summary

A study of the routine urinalysis was undertaken to determine the feasibility of automating the technique to achieve a degree of quantitation, accuracy, precision, sensitivity, specificity, rapidity, volume output and capability. Although there is considerable justification for extending the test battery, this feasibility study was designed to include only those tests currently included in the routine urinalysis: pH, protein, ketone bodies, color, glucose, hemoglobin, bilirubin and specific conductivity. Creatinine was incorporated as a means to allow more meaningful quantitation.

New and conventional chemical methods were adapted to modified continuous-flow automated systems. Primary standards, normal and pathologic specimens were analyzed. Normal ranges, precision, recovery and comparative data were compiled and analyzed.

The feasibility of automating urinalysis was proven. Quantitation of urine metabolites may be readily achieved. It appears reasonable that at some future time automated urine analysis will be routinely performed and that considerable patient benefit will accrue.

References

1. Feigle, F.: *Spot Tests In Organic Analysis.* New York:Elsevier Publishing Co., 1966.
2. *Detection and Prevention of Chronic Disease Utilizing Multiphasic Screening Techniques,* a report of the Subcommittee on Health of the Elderly to the Special Committee on Aging, U. S. Senate, 1966.
3. Lab growth keyed to computer revolution, editorial. *Lab World,* 19:1040-1042, 1968.
4. Pribor, H. D., Kirkham, W. R. and Hoyt, R. S.: Small computer does a big job in this hospital laboratory. *Mod. Hosp.,* 110:104-107, 1968.
5. Kark, R. M., Lawrence, J. R., Pottach, V. E. et al.: *A Primer of Urinalysis.* New York:Harper and Row, 1963.
6. Hepler, O. E.: Urinalysis. In Hepler, O. E. (ed.): *Manual of Clinical Laboratory Methods,* ed. 4. Springfield, Ill.:Charles C Thomas, 1963, pp. 3-32.
7. Hunter, D. T., Degn, V. and McGuire, L.: The assay of creatinine on the SMA-12. *Amer. J. Med. Techn.,* 34:405-407, 1968.
8. Peterson, J. I.: Urinary glucose measurement. *Clin. Chem.,* 14:513-520, 1968.
9. Rothera, A. C. H.: Note on the sodium nitro-prusside reaction for acetone. *J. Physiol.,* 37:491, 1908.
10. Henry, R. J.: Qualitative tests for protein. In Henry, R. J. (ed.): *Clinical Chemistry, Principles and Technics.* New York:Harper and Row, 1964, pp. 193-196.
11. Dubowski, K. M.: An O-toluidine method for body fluid glucose determination. *Clin. Chem.,* 8:215-235, 1962.
12. Oser, B. L.: Urine composition, quantitative analysis. In Oser, B. L. (ed.): *Hawk's Physiological Chemistry.* New York:McGraw-Hill Book Co. Inc., 1965, pp. 1152-1280.
13. Couch, R. D.: Routine screening for urinary bilirubin in hospitalized patients. *Amer. J. Clin. Path.,* 53:194-195, 1970.
14. Owen, J. A., Silberman, H. J. and Got, C.: Detection of haemoglobin, haemoglobin-haptoglobin complexes and other substances with peroxidase activity after zone electrophoresis. *Nature,* 182:1373. 1958.

Health Data Management: Ontario Plan

Donald J. Shepley

In Canada, the delivery of health care is primarily a provincial responsibility. Since it is impossible for the elected representatives to become completely conversant with all the details and aspects of the area for which he is responsible, a senior advisory body, The Ontario Council of Health, was established. One of the subcommittees of this group was charged with " . . . studying the role and potential use of computers in the health field and with developing recommendations relating to the distribution of different types of computers within the health facilities to best serve the population and for best utilization of the available computing capacity." A report was prepared and approved by the Council in January 1970.[1]

I participated in the preparation of the report to the Council and, therefore, I am able to give you some idea of the planning underway in Ontario (the items in quotes are taken from the report). Very quickly our group realized it was not the computer that had to be considered but rather, a "Health Information System," for the ultimate objective of the province in the area of application of computer technology to health care delivery must be the " . . . orderly development of a total health information system and that the primary orientation of the system be towards the needs of the individual citizen and not towards the needs of a health care facility, government agency, or other organizations." Further, we recommended that the system be based on " . . . the establishment of life-time personal health records for each provincial resident, and the establishment of derived and externally created banks of health related information."

The concept put forward by the Committee realized the tremendous complex of independent or autonomous entities and the staggering volumes of information with which a system would have to cope. The intent is such that each component in the complex can remain viable, usefully functional and autonomous, yet able to interact properly with the

Donald J. Shepley, M.D., *Director, Computer Systems, The Hospital for Sick Children, Toronto, Ontario, Canada.*

other components and still meet its own needs. Hence, the concept was put forward to structure information such that the details, wherever possible would be " . . . acquired, recorded and organized into an accessible form as close to the source or periphery as possible and that abstracts, or summaries, or key data be held within the network or system proper, with pointers to the files where the details would be kept." The major "systematized file," about which the system would revolve, would be the lifetime personal health records or what we titled the PDF (Personal Data File). Systematizing of personal information for dissemination to the providers of health care of course led to studies regarding what information should be available and to whom. To deal with this, recommendations were made that (1) " . . . all files of health related information wherever possible be made accessible to the system whether or not they are generated within the existing system of health care services," and (2) " . . . concurrent with the ultimate development of the total health information system every health facility, agency and individual participant where authorized, be provided access to the system."

Realizing the possible infringement of privacy and that the main feature of the system is the PDF, it was imperative to protect the privacy of individuals without inhibiting unnecessarily the potential for improving health care delivery, research and government planning. (It is of note that privacy only becomes a problem when the person can be identified through information released from the files.)

Unfortunately, there is no clear-cut way by which one may distinguish those who have access to personally identifiable information from those who may not. For this reason our committee proposed the establishment of a special group which would be concerned with rules and standards of access as well as appropriate legislation. Nonetheless, there were specific rules and standards which we recommended. These recommendations included a special group: " . . . the Privacy Committee be formed to deal with matters pertaining to access and disclosure of personal information with functions to include the following:

    a) definition of the level of access permitted to the different classes of users of the system,
    b) definitions of standards of disclosure of information,
    c) standardization of procedures of access and disclosure of information including a means of bypassing normal rules and restrictions in an emergency,
    d) provision of advice on the accreditation of qualified investigators for special research involving the disclosure of identity,
    e) provision of advice on the desirability of research involving the disclosure of identity,
    f) provision of advice on special requests not covered by established procedures."

We further recommended that:

1) "if an entity is to be preserved, access to information should be relatively simple and easy and that
2) physicians have access to the PDF of their patients and that
3) the written consent of his [the physician's] legal representative be obtained before information is disclosed to the research investigator; however, if the investigator provides adequate guarantees that he would use identifying information only for purposes acceptable to the Privacy Committee, for example, to link data between existing files for purposes of statistical analysis, and maintain the information so obtained in a manner acceptable to the Privacy Committee, then this procedure would be waived and that
4) rules and standards of disclosure be made known to the public,
5) that the individual have right of access of his own file to verify or modify it with the provision that
6) any modified or deleted item be flagged appropriately so long as flagging per se does not compromise the privacy of the individual
7) that all single unique non-statistical accession to the files be recorded in the PDF
8) that computer personnel working within the health information system be licensed."

I have only covered a few aspects briefly. Obviously, many more were considered in greater detail in the preparation of our plans. The implementation of such an approach requires definite plans, objectives and excellence of organization.

A subsequent report dealing with the steps towards implementation has recently been submitted to the Council but it is not yet published. I feel, however, practical and possible steps have been identified.

In summary, the need for organizing health information is great and the technology is present. The challenge now is for excellence in management.

Reference

1. *Health Care Delivery Systems – Role of Computers in the Health Field,* Report of the Ontario Council of Health, Supplement No. 9, 1970.